Psychology
in
Progress
General editor: Peter Herriot

Brain,
Behaviour
and Evolution

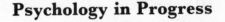

Psychology in Progress

Already available

Aspects of Memory
edited by Michael M. Gruneberg and Peter Morris

Thinking in Perspective
edited by Andrew Burton and John Radford

Issues in Childhood Social Development
edited by Harry McGurk

Philosophical Problems in Psychology
edited by Neil Bolton

Forthcoming

The School Years: A Social Psychological Perspective
edited by John Coleman

Brain, Behaviour and Evolution

edited by
DAVID A. OAKLEY
and
H. C. PLOTKIN

METHUEN

First published in 1979 by
Methuen & Co Ltd
11 New Fetter Lane London EC4P 4EE

This collection © Methuen & Co Ltd 1979
Individual chapters © the respective authors 1979

Filmset by Northumberland Press Ltd,
Gateshead, Tyne and Wear
and printed in Great Britain by
University Press Cambridge

ISBN   0 416 71260 6 (hardbound)
ISBN   0 416 71270 3 (paperback)

Contents

Notes on the contributors

Stuart Dimond is reader in psychology at University College, Cardiff. His research interests extend from animal behaviour to questions of hemisphere function of the human brain. He is the author of *Social Behaviour of Animals*, *The Double Brain*, *Hemisphere Function in the Human Brain* (edited with J. G. Beaumont), *Introducing Neuropsychology* and *Evolution and Lateralization of the Brain* (edited with D. A. Blizard). He has recently made a film called *Crossroads of the Brain* and is currently working on a book concerned with human brain function. He recently organized the Conference of the New York Academy of Sciences on 'Evolution and Lateralization of the Brain'.

Gaylord Ellison is Professor of Psychology at UCLA, Los Angeles, and a member of the Brain Research Institute and the Alcohol Research Center. From early studies in salivary conditioning in dogs, and effects of neural isolation of the hypothalamus on aggression and feeding behaviour in rats and cats, his research has gradually focused upon animal models of psychopathology. He is now studying hallucinatory behaviour and the permanent alterations in brain chemistry produced by amphetamine administration.

Ray Meddis is lecturer at the Department of Human Sciences,

University of Technology, Loughborough. While remaining interested in the theoretical aspects of the nature and function of sleep he has recently been working on the development of general rank sum tests in non-parametric statistical analysis. His publications include *Elementary Analysis of Variance for the Behavioural Sciences*, *Statistical Handbook for Non-statisticians* and *The Sleep Instinct*.

David A. Oakley lectures in psychology at University College London. He has published research on the role of neocortex in learning, on the maturation of locomotion and tonic immobility (animal hypnosis) in young mammals, and on aspects of learning theory, such as backward conditioning. He is currently interested in the physiological changes which follow neodecortication and in the evolutionary role of neocortex as it relates to sensory processes and imagery and to behaviour under semi-natural conditions. He is collaborating on a number of developmental, lesion and learning theory projects at University College London and The City University.

Linda Partridge lectures in zoology at the University of Edinburgh. Her research interests are in the area of overlap between population genetics, behaviour and ecology, and she has published papers on habitat selection and feeding behaviour in titmice and on social behaviour in birds and other animals. She has recently started work on the consequences of mate choice in fruitflies.

Henry Plotkin lectures in psychology at University College London. The award of an MRC travelling fellowship resulted in a period as a postdoctoral fellow at Stanford University, California, working with Professor K. H. Pribram, and he has also spent seven years as a scientific member of the MRC Unit on Neural Mechanisms of Behaviour. His research has always revolved around learning, which was initially pursued by way of physiological psychology but is now predominantly concerned with the development of learning, and with the relationship between learning, development and evolution. He is currently working on a number of mammalian developmental projects at University College London, and on learning in a species of predaceous ground beetle.

I. Steele Russell is Visiting Professor of Psychology at University College London and Director of the MRC Neural Mechanism of

Behaviour Unit. He is a member of the Executive Committee of the European Brain and Behaviour Society and Honourary Wetenschappelijk Hoofmedewerker in Physiology at the Erasmus University Medical School, Rotterdam. He is also the UK editor for *Physiology and Behaviour* and acts as scientific advisor in primatology at Rotterdam Zoo. His research interests include split-brain memory lateralization, decorticate learning, and the effects of frontal lobe lesion on behaviour.

Roger Wolcott Sperry is Hixon Professor of Psychobiology at the California Institute of Technology. His research interests range over a wide area of psychobiology, neuropsychology and neurobiology. He has published many experimental and review papers as well as articles and chapters in scientific journals and books. He is a member of the editorial boards of *Experimental Neurology*, *Experimental Brain Research*, *Neuropsychologia*, *The International Journal of Neuroscience*, *Behavioural Biology* and *Zygon*.

Christopher Yeo is presently studying interhemispheric and subcortical aspects of mammalian visual behaviour at the MRC Unit on Neural Mechanisms of Behaviour, University College London. His doctoral studies were an investigation of commissure function and the interhemispheric exchange of visual information in goldfish.

Editors' introduction

Evolutionary theory has revolutionized the biological sciences and our view of man in relation to other animals. Modern evolutionary theory also claims psychology and the social sciences as a branch of the biological sciences. It is a branch, however, which has not until very recently felt the full effect of the evolutionary approach and awaits inclusion in the post-Darwinian 'New Synthesis'. We believe that psychologists generally have much to gain, and really not much to lose, by listening to what evolutionary biologists have to say about their subject. Sleep, consciousness and freewill, for example, which are tackled in this volume, take on unaccustomed perspectives at the hands of biological theory. To achieve a synthesis of the sort implied above it is important that the psychologists involved should understand evolution. Unfortunately psychologists have frequently failed in this understanding. We have tried to correct some major misconceptions later in this introduction and we and the other authors have continued this process in the subsequent chapters. It is important also that the traffic of ideas between the biological sciences and psychology is not one-way and we hope that this volume will be of interest to students in zoology and related disciplines as well as to psychologists. This volume is called *Brain, Behaviour and Evolution*. Psychology is represented by 'Behaviour' and we have stated our belief in the importance of 'Evolution'. The 'Brain' stands for the central nervous system, which serves as a major link between evolution and behaviour.

An evolutionary approach to psychology encourages us to see human behaviour, from the eye-blink reflex to complex cognitive activity, as examples of adaptive behaviours whose significance can best be evaluated in relation to similar phenomena in other animals. Many human activities, such as sleeping, feeding, fighting, reproducing, perceiving, learning, remembering and socializing, we know from observation are shared by other animals. Others, such as language, consciousness, freewill and forward planning we have tended to regard as purely human attributes. Evolutionary theory challenges this easy assumption on the grounds of continuity of the evolutionary process. There is no good evolutionary reason to suppose, for example, that consciousness is limited to man (see Chapters 7 and 9).

To take just one example of the application of evolutionary reasoning to an unresolved problem in psychology, that of the function of sleep (see Chapter 5), an evolutionary theorist might argue as follows: as the majority of vertebrates show the characteristic phenomenon of sleep it is parsimonious to commence an explanation of the function of sleep in the simplest terms which will account for its presence wherever it is found rather than to begin with purely human interpretations. Whilst it is true that some aspects of human sleep function may eventually be shown to be species specific it is unlikely that sleep evolved in the first place to resolve psychodynamic tensions, alleviate neurosis or to process the residues of complex cognitive activities as some theories of human sleep propose. If he were to adopt the role of Devil's Advocate our evolutionary theorist might further suggest that the original and perhaps only function of sleep (as part of a behavioural device for staying out of the way of nocturnal predators for example) is no longer applicable to man. He could then conclude that human sleep represents a purely useless evolutionary vestige which, as it is not actually detrimental, natural selection has not eliminated. If the latter were true human sleep would be explicable *only* in evolutionary terms and any attempt to explain its current function in man would clearly be doomed to failure. A view stated in such extreme terms would win our theorist few friends among human sleep researchers, though in the absence of any convincing demonstration of the function of sleep in man his views would be difficult to refute. Whatever the resolution of this particular question there seems to us to be considerable merit in considering first the general significance of sleep, or any other behaviour, for all animals, and only then to consider any purely human functions it might have if the former account is found incomplete for man. Similarly we might consider consciousness not as a human luxury, a television screen into brain activity, but as an evolved process which increases chances of survival in man and which may serve the same survival functions in other animals, especially those with brains similar to our own. Evolutionary theory suggests new, and we believe productive, ways of looking at traditional problems in psychology.

In fact the need for an interdisciplinary approach is increasingly accepted and biological studies of behaviour (that is, studies whose basic assumptions, tenets and models are rooted in one or other of the biological sciences such as genetics, ecology or physiology) are appearing at an unprecedented and accelerating rate. Any single volume, and a slim one at that, which seeks to review the subject must be highly selective. Other editors would have chosen different topics and used different authors and so it is well to say why this volume takes the form it does.

The chapters are of two types. Those which supply basic information and those which are expositions on particular topics. The former are intended to supply elementary knowledge concerning evolutionary theory and genetics (Chapter 1), the structure and morphology of the vertebrate nervous system (Chapter 2) and the relationship between evolutionary and process biology (Chapter 3). The remaining chapters are reviews of behavioural and psychological areas where both evolutionary and neurological perspectives can be applied. We hope that by supplying both background information as well as the subject expositions the volume will be relatively self-contained. The student should, however, be aware that the information contained in Chapters 1 and 2 is necessarily restricted. Chapter 1, for example, is quite literally an introduction to the evolution and genetics of behaviour. The readings that the author suggests at the end of the chapter are almost as important as the chapter contents themselves. As all behaviour is a product of processes occurring in different parts of the central nervous system we believe that students of psychology should have some knowledge of traditional neuroanatomy (Chapter 2) and that a developmental and comparative approach makes the acquisition of such knowledge easier. We suspect that psychology students find both these areas difficult to handle if they are asked to go away and read them in separate sources. Hence our including simplified accounts of them in this volume. We also believe that far too little is written about, and hence far too few students think about, how the two great subdivisions of behavioural biology are related to one another, which accounts for Chapter 3.

Chapter 4 introduces the newly discovered chemical systems of the brain and reviews the behavioural effects of some of them in relation to the varying demands of natural environments. The remaining five subject-expository chapters follow a single theme. This is our increasing knowledge of the vertebrate forebrain, especially in birds and mammals, and how its evolution appears to relate to such areas as learning, memory, intelligence, complex-problem solving, cross-modal integration, reasoning, consciousness, freewill, sleep and dreaming. We felt that our selectivity should have some thematic unity, and this was our choice. The price, of course, has been paid. There is little in this volume on motivation and drive, perception, motor processes and skills. Perhaps if the publishers pursue this series to a second stage then these are some of the topics that will be included next time around.

There is one issue which we want to clarify here because it has plagued us throughout the editing of this text and, indeed, has been a constant thorn in the flesh of comparative studies of brain and behaviour for a long time. This is the problem of how one orders animals and of choosing the descriptive labels that are used in comparing different animals. Traditionally psychology has employed the notion of a phylogenetic scale which places single celled creatures at one end (the bottom) and man at the other (the top), with worms, fish, rats and monkeys appropriately ordered in between. The phylogenetic scale (or *scala naturae*), however, is one of the great myths of modern science. It is a wholly invalid conceptualization of life, both taxonomically and functionally (Hodos and Campbell, 1969; Lockard, 1971). Psychology is slowly coming to realize it, and most biologists know it. None the less, even the most eminent biologists are apt to slip into usage of 'higher' and 'lower' or 'advanced' and 'primitive', and even if it is not intended, the reader is inclined to interpret such labels as congruent with a phylogenetic scale. Virtually every author in this volume has had to employ such descriptive labels and we have tried to standardize the usage.

We have eliminated higher–lower on the authority of no less a figure than Darwin himself, who warned against the anthropocentrism inherent in such terminology. Complex–simple is also a particularly poor scale. First, it implies a directional change in time from the more simple to the increasingly complex across one or several functional attributes and there is simply no evidence to support such an implication. Second, it has frequently been used to imply 'progress' in evolutionary change. Williams (1966) has argued effectively against the notion of generalized progress as being biological nonsense at worst, or misguided anthropocentrism at best – there is no reason to doubt man's cognitive supremacy, but equally there is no reason to assume that evolution has been progressing towards such a preordained goal. Third, complexity or competence in terms of one attribute does not mean complexity or competence in all attributes. Man is not very good in water, and there may be equally misguided ichthiocentric fish who consider man a rather lowly creature.

Advanced–primitive tends again to have anthropocentric overtones. Yet it also has something in common with more evolved/less evolved and more differentiated/less differentiated, and in general we have tended to favour the latter. This is because we think that the most sensible scale of comparison relates to the extent to which the animals being compared differ from their common ancestor, no matter how remote in time each is from that ancestor. For example, while it is nonsense to describe a salmon (a teleost or 'bony' fish) as being lower or more simple than a chimpanzee (a placental mammal), it is reasonable to assume that the salmon is both morphologically and behaviourally more like the archaic jawed fishes (the placoderms) than is the chimpanzee. In Figure 1 the placoderms would appear around 400 million years ago close to the point where the teleost and elasmobranch branches leave the main evolutionary tree and thus form the common ancestry of modern teleost fish as well as mammals like the chimpanzee. Thus we consider the salmon to be a less differentiated form than the chimpanzee because we think that the former has changed less over time than the latter *relative to their common ancestry*. The chimpanzee, for example, possesses features such as homeothermy and the ability to live on dry land, both of which are features which evolved later in geological time, after the basic pattern of aquatic vertebrates had emerged. There is no place in such scales, however, for value-laden terms such as higher or more progressive. It should also be noted that we use the term differentiation in its common English usage and not as embryologists use it.

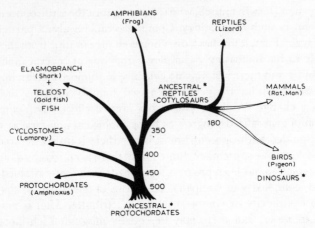

Fig. 1   Simplified plan of the evolutionary history of the major classes of modern vertebrates. Living examples of each class are shown in brackets. Open arrows indicate homeothermic (warm-blooded) classes. Black arrows indicate poikilothermic (cold-blooded)classes. * = extinct. Numbers = time (in millions of years) before the present. Arrow heads = present day. The direction of branching (to left or right) on this representation is arbitrary.

There is some justification also, on the basis of palaeontological evidence, for saying that aquatic vertebrates evolved before amphibians, amphibians before reptiles, and reptiles before birds and mammals. On this basis fish (which represent the early aquatic vertebrate niche) can be said to represent an early evolved group and mammals a later evolved group. By the same token, however, the modern fish have had exactly the same amount of time (400 million years) to diverge from their common ancestor as have all the later vertebrates. Some fishes have diverged more than others. The brain of teleost fish, for example, appears to be vastly different from that of its placoderm ancestor whereas the elasmobranch ('cartiloginous') fish brain has changed less in its gross anatomy. As a result the brain of a descendant of an even earlier offshoot from the common vertebrate stock, such as the lamprey, may better represent the ancestral fish brain.

Figure 2 places the modern mammals within the context of a restricted phylogenetic tree. We have quite deliberately placed the major placental orders in alphabetical sequence from left to right. The rat should no more be considered higher than man than man should be considered higher than the rabbit. They are simply different

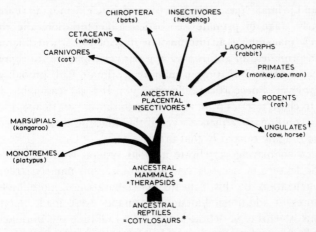

Fig. 2 Simplified plan of the evolutionary history of the major orders of modern mammals. Mammals may be roughly characterized as warm-blooded animals, usually covered with fur or hair, whose young are suckled by the female with milk produced in specialized (mammary) glands. Of the ten orders of modern mammals shown in this figure, the monotremes produce their young inside a large, shelled egg, and in this respect are the least differentiated of the mammals. The young of marsupials are born alive but as very immature embryos, which are then usually transferred to a protective pouch (marsupium). The other eight orders are placental mammals which retain their young within the mother's body where they are brought to an advanced stage of embryological development by means of a nutritive placenta. Living examples of each order are shown in brackets. The modern placental mammals are shown in alphabetical order. * = extinct. † = strictly speaking a collection of orders.

from one another. It is possible to scale them again on the basis of their difference from a common ancestral form but to do so it is necessary to specify precisely the dimension along which the differentiation has taken place. In a comparison of neocortical expansion, for instance, it is probably reasonable to suggest that modern insectivores have changed rather little from the common insectivore stock, the rodents and lagomorphs have changed more, whilst carnivores and primates show the greatest neocortical development. It is essential to remember though that all have done so along their separate phylogenetic paths. It may be reasonable, for instance, to erect a quasi-evolutionary series which comprises a modern insectivore (e.g. hedgehog) to represent the ancestral placental stock, the modern tree shrew (*Tupaia glis*) to represent the transition between insecti-

vore and primate lines, a modern prosimian (e.g. lemur) to represent
an early stage of primate neocortical differentiation, the rhesus
monkey (macaque) as an intermediate stage of neocortical differentiation in primates, an anthropoid ape (e.g. chimpanzee) to represent
a later stage, culminating in man as a primate with probably the
highest level of neocortical differentiation. It is *not* reasonable, however, to claim a series from insectivore to rat, to cat, to ape, to man
as an evolutionary sequence, even if the differentiation of neocortex
can be roughly ranked in that order.

When comparing vertebrate nervous systems we have chosen a
specific feature of nervous system organization, namely structural
encephalization. By this is meant the elaboration of more forebrain
structures as additional functional demands were made upon the
nervous systems of vertebrates who were radiating out into increasingly diverse and demanding ecological niches (see Jerison, 1976).

Throughout this volume, therefore, we have tried to standardize the
terminology of comparisons between animals to either more or less
differentiated when the writer is being general, to early and later
evolved when the perspective is historical and to more or less
encephalized when the writer is referring specifically to neurological
comparisons between vertebrates.

DAVID OAKLEY

H. C. PLOTKIN

References

Hodos, W. and Campbell, C. B. G. (1969) Scala naturae: why there is no
theory in comparative psychology. *Psychological Review 76*: 337–50.

Jerison, H. J. (1976) Principles of the evolution of the brain and behaviour.
In R. B. Masterton, W. Hodos and H. Jerison (eds.) *Evolution, Brain and
Behaviour: Persistent Problems*. Hillsdale, New Jersey: Lawrence Erlbaum,
23–45.

Lockard, R. B. (1971) Reflections on the fall of comparative psychology: Is
there a message for us all? *American Psychologist 26*: 168–79.

Williams, G. C. (1966) *Adaptation and Natural Selection*. Princeton, New Jersey:
Princeton University Press.

1   The evolution and genetics of behaviour[1]

Linda Partridge

Introduction

Darwin's theory of evolution through natural selection is the main
unifying idea in biology today. In this respect the development of
psychology has proceeded rather separately from that of biology. It
has always concentrated upon man, and usually the comparative
approach has not been used to study the evolution of behaviour, but
in the hope that 'animals' will act as simplified types of human beings.
Certainly there are some respects in which mechanisms basic to the
organization of all behaviour can be best studied in animals. However,
we lose a whole dimension of animal behaviour if we ignore its diverse
origins and the selective forces which shaped it.

Animal behaviour is often known as comparative psychology in
psychology departments, and as ethology in biology departments.
Although they sometimes deal with similar subject matter, these two
approaches have very different histories and aims. Comparative psychology takes place in the laboratory, and has traditionally been concerned with 'intelligence', problem-solving abilities and other mental
traits in animals. Most of the studies have used the laboratory rat.
These studies were based upon the idea of a phylogenetic scale of
intelligence with 'lowly' animals at the bottom, man at the top, and

rats and monkeys somewhere in between. One central assumption which has been made by comparative psychologists is that learning is the key to animal behaviour because most behaviour is acquired, and that because so little is built into animals, genetics and evolution are irrelevant to psychology.

Ethology, in contrast, is closely linked with genetics, evolution and ecology, and is the study of animal behaviour as an evolved character. In this approach both learned and inherited behaviour traits are studied in the context of the natural history of the animal. Rather than viewing the different behaviours and skills of different species as part of a phylogenetic scale of intelligence, ethologists consider that present-day species are evolved derivatives of ancestral forms which underwent diversification into many different species, which have become highly ecologically specialized. Every species has an aggregate of special abilities, each of which evolved as a response to ecological factors posing problems. Part of every animal's repertoire is inherited, and for this reason the study of genetics is seen as highly relevant to animal behaviour.

These two approaches are much less separate than they used to be, and each has made useful contributions to the other. There is now little doubt that behaviour has evolved, and that both genetically determined differences between animals in how they behave, and differences in the context and extent of learning, can be understood in the light of ecological differences.

In this chapter an outline of current views on evolution and genetics will be given especially as they apply to behaviour including human behaviour. The application of evolutionary and genetic ideas to social behaviour will then be discussed.

The theory of evolution by natural selection

What follows is a brief outline of Darwin's theory of natural selection. An excellent introduction to the subject is given by Maynard Smith (1975), and a more advanced account by Dobzhansky et al. (1977).

The clearest way to explain the theory is probably to give an account of the development of Darwin's own ideas. When in 1831 he set off for his voyage on HMS *Beagle*, Darwin was already aware of many of the facts which eventually contributed to his theory. In the eighteenth century Linnaeus had introduced his classification of the known species of animals and plants. Linnaeus viewed species as fixed entities, members of the same species having a characteristic morphology which was different from that of other species. He grouped together species in a hierarchical classification, a process called taxonomy. His system is still used today. In it, for example, man is a member of the Family Hominidae (which includes fossil men as well as modern man), the Order Primates (which includes monkeys and apes), the Class Mammalia (which includes cows, hedgehogs, lions and dolphins), the Subphylum Vertebrata (which includes fish, frogs, reptiles, birds and mammals) and the Phylum Chordata (which includes all animals with a stiff rod or spine, the notochord, running along the length of the body). In his classification Linnaeus recognized that animals and plants fall naturally into groups resembling one another in a variety of respects. The whales, for example, could be classified as fish on the grounds that they live in water and are streamlined. However, unlike fish and in common with mammals they have warm blood, a four-chambered heart, a characteristic arrangement of the skeletal bones and other internal organs, and they suckle their young with mammary glands. The fact that species can be grouped on the basis of resemblance in many respects could imply either that species were created as variations on a number of themes, or instead that their similarities were caused by descent from common ancestors. Linnaeus himself believed in separate creation, and thought that he was uncovering the design of the creator in making his classification. In contrast, several biologists before Darwin held evolutionary views, believing that all living creatures are descended from one or a few ancestors, and that similar forms have a more recent common ancestor than those that have less in common. By implication such an evolutionary outlook would view species as changing entities.

Darwin was also aware that animals and plants are adapted to their environments. Animals which live in cold areas have special means of insulation, such as thick coats of fur or layers of fat below the skin. Some, such as the mountain hare, turn white in winter and are camouflaged against the snowy background. They turn brown again in spring at about the time the snow melts. Camouflage as a defence against predators is a common phenomenon in animals, examples of dramatic cases being the resemblance of some moths to dead leaves, and of other insects to twigs. Some harmless insects are similar in appearance and behaviour to poisonous forms or to species with stings and are hence protected against predation.

The occurrence of adaptation is particularly obvious both when members of distantly related species come to resemble one another because they live in similar environments (the similarity in form of whales and fish is an example), and when members of related species become different in form because of differences in habits. Moles and bats are both modern mammals derived from the insectivore stock. Moles burrow in the ground and their fore-limbs are modified to form powerful shovels, while the fore-limbs of bats are modified to form wings. Adaptation has been thought to imply design by a creator.

When Darwin visited South America he was particularly impressed by the fossilized animal remains which he found there. Many of them, for example the bones of the giant sloths and armadillos, belonged to species which had become extinct, but which closely resembled much smaller modern counterparts. Others, such as fossil horses, have died out altogether, since there were no horses in South America when the Spaniards arrived there in the sixteenth century. In his diary Darwin commented : 'This wonderful resemblance between the dead and the living will, I do not doubt, hereafter throw much light on the appearance of organic beings on earth and their disappearance from it.' He also speculated that the extinct species might have died out because of their failure to adjust to their environment. At about that time the geologists William Smith and Charles Lyell both showed that successions of fossils in rock strata gave evidence of continuous change of form through geological time.

Darwin's views were crystallised by his visit to the Galapagos Islands, a group of volcanic islands in the Pacific some 600 miles west of Ecuador. He found that on several of the islands there existed giant tortoises, and that it was possible to tell from which island any particular tortoise came by the shape of its shell. This led Darwin to speculate that the different island forms, while still members of the same species, had diverged when geographically isolated from each other. Living on the islands Darwin also found a group of finches, now known as Darwin's finches, consisting of fourteen very similar species. The finches are confined to the Galapagos, and they differ from each other in their bill shapes and feeding methods. Some have heavy bills and eat large seeds, others have more slender bills and eat smaller seeds, some eat insects and one feeds on nectar. There are few other land birds on the Galapagos, and the finches occupy between them a number of niches which on the mainland would be occupied by other birds such as thrushes, woodpeckers, warblers and so on. Darwin remarked: 'Seeing this gradation and diversity of structure in one small, intimately related group of birds one might really fancy that from an original paucity of birds in this archipelago one species had been taken and modified for different ends.' He speculated that the different species had diverged in a similar way to the giant tortoises while in isolation on different islands, and that when dispersal resulted in two divergent forms coming together on one island they had changed so much that they would not interbreed, and had in fact become two species.

When he returned to England Darwin encountered two further ideas which were important for his theory. The first of these was contained in Malthus' 'Essay on Population', in which he argued, on the basis of human fecundity, that the human population is capable of increasing indefinitely in geometric progression. Since human populations do not increase in this way, Malthus argued, they must be held in check by the limited amount of food available. There is still little evidence that the main factor holding the human population in check was food, but the observation that animal and plant species are capable of indefinite increase in numbers under favourable conditions was important in Darwin's theory.

Lastly, Darwin was impressed by the changes which could be brought about by selective breeding of domestic animals. Again, this suggested to him that species were not immutable and could be modified by selective breeding of particular varieties.

Darwin went on to argue that since animals do not increase indefinitely in numbers, it follows that not all individuals survive to sexual maturity, or that some sexually mature individuals do not breed, or that breeding individuals produce fewer offspring than they would under optimal circumstances. Not all individuals in a species are alike, and at least some differences between them will affect their chances of survival and their fertility. In the ensuing struggle for existence some individuals will be better adapted than others to survive and reproduce and these will leave more offspring. This process is called natural selection. If the characteristics which enabled their parents to survive and reproduce are transmitted to the offspring, there will be evolution of characters bringing about adaptation. Thus by the combined processes of natural selection and of inheritance, the adaptation of the population to its environment is continuously maintained or improved, or is adjusted to a changing environment. An important aspect of Darwin's theory was that he believed that the hereditary variations upon which selection acted were in their origin non-adaptive. However at that time virtually nothing was known about the basis of heredity, and it was therefore doubted that such random non-adaptive hereditary variations could occur. This is discussed further in the next section.

Darwin's theory was greeted with uproar for two reasons. First, it conflicted with the account of the creation of living things given in the Book of Genesis. Second, it implied that man himself was the result of natural selection acting upon random hereditary variations in ape-like ancestors.

Since Darwin's death an enormous amount of work has been done in the fields of comparative anatomy, comparative embryology, population biology and genetics, and this work has yielded further support for the theory.

So far the evolution of the physical structure of animals has been discussed. Part of the structure of many animals is their nervous system, which is partly responsible for determining how they behave. There is now abundant evidence that behaviour can be adaptive in the same way as any other characteristic. One very elegant study of the adaptiveness of behaviour was carried out by Cullen (1957). She was studying a cliff-nesting seabird, the kittiwake, and found that in comparison with other species of gulls, which nest on flat ground, the kittiwake has certain behavioural peculiarities that adapt it to cliff nesting. Predation is less on cliffs than on flat ground, so that kittiwakes give fewer alarm calls and show less anti-predator behaviour such as the removal of conspicuous broken eggshells after the young have hatched. Parent kittiwakes do not recognize their chicks individually at least up to the age of four weeks, probably because the chicks cannot stray from the ledge. Ground-nesting gulls recognize their young a few days after hatching, and their chicks stray from the nest at an early age. Kittiwake nests are made of mud so that they stick to the rock ledges, while those of other gulls are made of grasses, mosses and other such materials. There are also differences in the aggressive and courtship displays, associated with the inability of young kittiwakes to leave the ledge in the face of aggression from strange adults, and with the cramped conditions on the ledges where courtship occurs.

There is also evidence that behaviour has evolved with other features in the formation of groups and species, so that it can be used as a character in taxonomy. Lorenz has used behaviour as a character in the taxonomy of ducks and geese. Any behaviour which is to be used as a taxonomic character must be present in all members of a species and it must be inherited. Lorenz has used various behaviours of young ducks and geese, and some of the aggressive and courtship displays of the adults as the basis of a classification. Behaviours which many species share are assumed to have evolved early in the formation of the group, while a behaviour which is present in only one species is assumed to have evolved after the separation of that species from the others. The use of behaviour resulted in several modifications to the classification of the ducks and geese.

It is rare to be able to see natural selection in action, but some examples have been produced by the activities of man. One example is the phenomenon of industrial melanism. One of the effects of industrial air pollution is to cause a darkening of tree trunks in the woods in industrial areas, both because soot is deposited and because gaseous pollution kills the pale lichens which grow on bark. Since the industrial revolution many species of moth which were previously pale in colour and were camouflaged on the tree bark have evolved dark colouration because of the spread of mutations causing dark colour. These dark moths are better camouflaged against the darkened bark than were the pale varieties and hence less likely to be eaten by birds. This change in colour has been accompanied by a change in the background selection by the moths. In the peppered moth a pale variety occurs in unpolluted rural areas while a dark form occurs in urban areas. If these two varieties are given a choice of white and black backgrounds on which to rest, the dark variety usually picks the black background, while the pale form usually selects the white background. Natural selection has here not only acted on mutations affecting the colour of the moths, but has also affected their background choice.

The extent to which learning occurs, and what can or cannot be learnt, is adaptive. Certain elements of behaviour seem not to be learned in that they appear in their usual form the first time a particular situation is encountered. A male fruitfly of a certain age will court the first female he encounters without having practised or observed other males courting. Thus apparently unlearned behaviour may be associated with situations where it can be predicted, far in advance, what the appropriate behaviour should be. For example, a male fruitfly should always court any female he encounters since his contribution to the next generation will depend greatly on how many females he inseminates. In contrast, young chicks learn the appearance of their own mother during the first few hours of life, and it would not be possible for this recognition to occur in any other way.

There are constraints on which responses can be elicited by particular stimuli during learning. For example, rats can learn to avoid a light or sound if it is associated with an electric shock, but not if it is associated with a taste cue. On the other hand, they can learn to avoid a taste which is associated with a poison, but not a sound or light which is associated with a poison. In terms of the rat's natural history this makes sense. In the wild, a poison is likely to be introduced in plant food, and hence would usually be associated with taste cues, while unpleasant sensations in the skin are likely to be paired with events outside the rat which might be associated with particular sights or sounds.

Darwin applied this theory to the evolution of man and human behaviour. He argued that there is no fundamental difference between man and the higher animals in their mental faculties, but he was also aware of the special roles which culture and language must have played in the evolution of human societies.

The mechanism of inheritance

Introduction

Our everyday experience tells us that offspring tend to resemble their parents. At the grossest level this is apparent from the fact that species breed true, but within species too we can see heredity at work. Within a human population tall parents tend on average to have taller offspring than do short parents. Several hereditary diseases are known in humans. Diabetes is inherited, although the exact mechanism is uncertain, and haemophilia, a disease which causes its sufferers to bleed profusely when cut, is also inherited.

We have seen in the previous section that natural selection acting on hereditary variation causes evolution. I will now describe some of the experiments which have contributed to current views on the mechanism of inheritance. An excellent introduction to this subject is given by Srb et al. (1965).

Lamarckism

Darwin speculated at some length about how inheritance might work, but he did not live to learn any of the answers. Towards the end of his life Darwin came to believe the ideas of Lamarck. Lamarck said that modifications of structures brought about by their use and disuse during the life of an animal were transmitted to the offspring. According to this hypothesis the evolution of the long neck of the giraffe would be explained by suggesting that the ancestors of modern giraffes started stretching their necks in order to reach the food supply in trees. The slight elongation of the neck which resulted was transmitted to the offspring at the time of reproduction. Presumably the accumulation of changes of this sort would gradually alter the characteristics of the species. Lamarck was not the first to think that changes acquired in this manner could be transmitted to the next generation, but he crystallized and popularized the notion and it has come to be called Lamarckism.

Many experiments have been done in an attempt to test Lamarck's ideas. For instance, Pavlov tried to show that the results of conditioning mice were inherited. He trained mice to respond to a bell which was sounded before every occasion on which food arrived. He counted the number of trials necessary to train the parents, bred from them, and repeated the process with their offspring, looking for an increase in the speed with which they learnt to respond. His results were negative, there being no improvement with time.

Lamarck's ideas have in general not been supported by experimental evidence (but for some contrary findings see Koestler, 1971) and are not accepted by scientists today.

Blending inheritance

Darwin eventually believed in the inheritance of acquired characteristics (Lamarckism) because of his inability to deal with one major objection to his earlier beliefs about the mechanism of inheritance. That mechanism, known as blending inheritance, was based on the assumption that the characteristics of offspring were a half-and-half mixture of all the characteristics of their two parents. Assuming that an individual with a new useful variation arises in the population and mates with a normal partner, its offspring would inherit only 50 per cent of the useful new feature, its grandchildren 25 per cent and so on. Eventually the useful variation would disappear. Such a mechanism seems highly unlikely to give rise to evolutionary change. Darwin was unaware that in 1865 the answer to this problem was published by Gregor Mendel, an Augustinian monk living in Brunn, Moravia. Mendel's paper was rediscovered in 1900.

Major genes

Mendel worked on pea plants in the garden of the monastery. His experiments involved crossing different varieties of peas and noting the appearance of the offspring. He investigated seven characteristics in all, and his results for each characteristic were the same.

In one of his experiments Mendel crossed a tall pea with a dwarf variety. In the first generation of offspring (called the F_1) all of the plants were tall. In all of his seven crosses with contrasting characters only one parental characteristic appeared in the F_1 and that characteristic was said to be *dominant* to the alternative character which was said to be *recessive*. Mendel then made crosses between two of his F_1 plants. In their offspring, the F_2 generation, plants showing the dominant trait and plants showing the recessive trait were both found among the offspring in an approximate ratio of 3 tall to 1 dwarf. No plants were intermediate. Furthermore, if the dwarf plants were self-pollinated (mated to themselves) they bred true and produced only dwarf offspring. One third of the tall plants also bred true when self-pollinated, but two thirds again gave progeny in a ratio of 3 tall to 1 dwarf.

To account for these results Mendel suggested that each parent possessed two elements which determined the particular trait. Each parent transmitted *only one* of its two elements to an offspring, and each element was equally likely to be transmitted. If the parents differed in a characteristic, an element contributed by one parent might be dominant over that contributed by the other parent, and then the offspring would resemble the first parent. None the less, the recessive element, although not visible, would not be destroyed or contaminated in any way by its association with the dominant element. When the individual bred it would pass on the elements that it had received from each parent to half its progeny, because one element would be transmitted half the time and the alternative element the rest of the time.

If the tall plant used by Mendel had two elements for tallness called T, so that it was TT, while the dwarf plant had two elements for dwarfness tt, then Mendel's crosses can be represented as in Figure 1.1.

Mendel's elements are now called genes, and the study of their transmission is called genetics. Alternative elements such as T and t are said to be *alleles* of the same gene. Genes are passed from one generation to the next in cells called *gametes*, and the genes are carried in these cells in linear arrays in bodies called *chromosomes* which are visible with a microscope. Alleles which are carried on the same chromosome tend to go together into the gametes and are said to be linked, but genes which are on different chromosomes are distributed independently. Gametes contain half as many chromosomes as the other cells of the body. In humans the gametes contain 23 chromosomes while the cells in, for example, the liver or the brain contain 23 *pairs* of chromosomes. If an individual carries two different alleles of a contrasting pair such as, in man, the allele causing brown eyes and that causing blue eyes, then the allele for one character is carried on one of the relevant pair of chromosomes, while the allele for the contrasting character is carried on the other. Individuals carrying the same two alleles, such as Mendel's tt plants are called *homozygotes*, while his Tt plants, with two different alleles, are called *heterozygotes*. Another important distinction is between the overt characteristics of an individual, called its *phenotype*, and the genes which it contains, constituting its *genotype*. For example, TT and Tt plants have different genotypes but the same phenotype (tall).

Mutation

If genes are unaffected by their sojourn in a particular individual, then how do new hereditary variations ever arise? It seems that genes are made of a chemical which can undergo discrete changes, called mutations, which alter the structure of the gene and may alter the phenotype to which it gives rise. Mutation occurs naturally at a very low rate, but its incidence can be greatly increased by irradiation with X-rays and by certain chemical mutagens. An important characteristic of naturally occurring mutations is that they are random in respect of the current needs of the animal. A mutation causing a mouse to grow a thicker coating of hair is no more likely to occur in a cold environment than in a hot one. These random mutations are the raw material for natural selection.

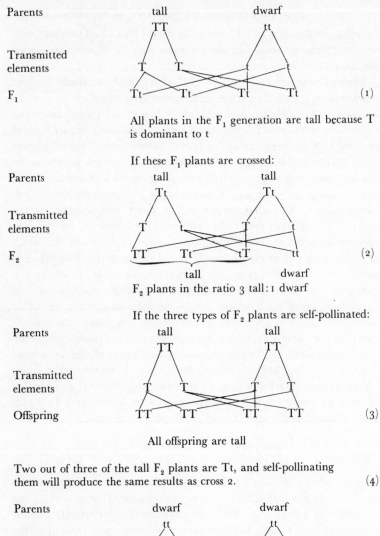

Parents   tall   dwarf

TT   tt

Transmitted elements

T   T   t   t

F_1 Tt   Tt   Tt   Tt   (1)

All plants in the F_1 generation are tall because T is dominant to t

If these F_1 plants are crossed:

Parents   tall   tall

Tt   Tt

Transmitted elements

T   t   T   t

F_2 TT   Tt   tT   tt   (2)

tall   dwarf

F_2 plants in the ratio 3 tall : 1 dwarf

If the three types of F_2 plants are self-pollinated:

Parents   tall   tall

TT   TT

Transmitted elements

T   T   T   T

Offspring   TT   TT   TT   TT   (3)

All offspring are tall

Two out of three of the tall F_2 plants are Tt, and self-pollinating them will produce the same results as cross 2.   (4)

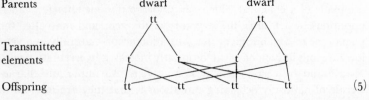

Parents   dwarf   dwarf

tt   tt

Transmitted elements

t   t   t   t

Offspring   tt   tt   tt   tt   (5)

All offspring are dwarf

Fig. 1.1   Mendel's crosses. (1) A cross between a tall and a dwarf plant. (2) A cross between two of the tall F_1 plants. (3), (4) and (5) Self-pollination of the three classes of F_2 plants.

Continuous variation

Given a number of individuals of the same genotype, we might none the less expect phenotypic differences among them caused by environmental agents. An example of this is height in man, where both heredity and nutrition affect adult height. We cannot, except arbitrarily, categorize humans into discrete height classes because height is a continuously varying character. This is partly because it is affected by nutrition so that genetic effects are blurred, but it is also because more than one pair of genes affects height. Where several different non-allelic genes affect one character, it is then said to be under polygenic control and in general the more genes involved, the more continuous is the variation observed. How can the intrinsically discontinuous variation caused by genes be expressed as continuous variation?

Suppose that an individual of genotype Aa Bb (A is dominant to its allele a, and B is dominant to b, and the two genes are on different chromosomes and are transmitted independently) is crossed with another of identical genotype. The alleles A and B increase height by one unit, while the alternatives a and b decrease it by one unit. The results of the cross are shown in Figure 1.2. It can be seen that the F_1 progeny fall into five height categories, and it is fairly easy to see that if more genes were involved the observed distribution of height would rapidly become continuous, especially if environmental influences were also involved.

The study of the genetics underlying continuous variation is more complicated than for major genes. Several different techniques are used. Some involve the use of inbred strains, made by many generations of mating of brothers to sisters so that the animals become genetically homozygous. All variation within inbred strains should be caused by environment, while variation between inbred strains of the same species reared and tested in identical environments is genetic, different alleles having become fixed (homozygous) in the different strains. In humans, monozygotic twins have the same genotype, so that differences between them are likely to be environmental in origin.

Another method used for both humans and animals is to examine the similarities between different classes of relatives, e.g. siblings, first cousins and so on. Close relatives are likely to hold more genes in common by descent than are more distant relatives or members of

Parents   AaBb   AaBb

A and a are transmitted to the gametes independently of B and b so that all four combinations are equally likely

Gametes   AB Ab aB ab   AB Ab aB ab

F_1

	AB	Ab	aB	ab
AB	+4 AABB	+2 AABb	+2 aABB	0 aAbB
Ab	+2 AABb	0 AAbb	0 aABb	−2 aAbb
aB	+2 AaBB	0 AabB	0 aaBB	−2 aabB
ab	0 AaBb	−2 Aabb	−2 aaBb	−4 aabb

Above each F_1 offspring is written its net height score where:
A = B = + 1
a = b = − 1

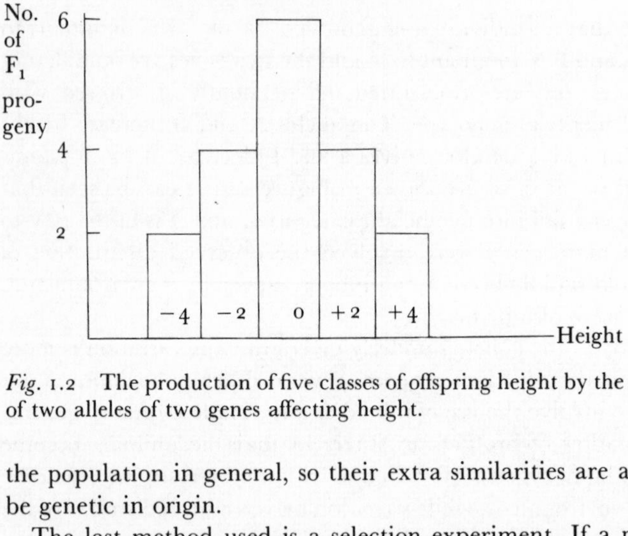

No. of F_1 progeny

Fig. 1.2   The production of five classes of offspring height by the segregation of two alleles of two genes affecting height.

the population in general, so their extra similarities are assumed to be genetic in origin.

The last method used is a selection experiment. If a population varies in respect of a character such as size, then if the variation is genetic in origin a mating between two large individuals should produce progeny which on average are larger than those produced by a mating between two small individuals. This process can be repeated for many generations. Such experiments have shown that there is genetic variation for an enormous number of characters in animal populations.

Cultural inheritance

For natural selection to act there must be hereditary variation in the character being selected. Some variation in behaviour is achieved by one generation learning from its parents or other individuals, a process called cultural inheritance. The role of cultural traditions in causing differences between human populations is enormous, and it also occurs in animals. One example concerns the transmission of feeding behaviour in monkeys, where in a group of Japanese macaques (monkeys) one individual started to wash her food before she ate it. This habit gradually spread to the rest of the troop as a result of imitation. Another example concerns the opening of milk bottles by birds in Britain. Great tits in several areas learned to peck through the foil caps on milk bottles, and the habit spread rapidly, almost certainly too fast for natural selection of a mutation to have been involved. Cultural inheritance is also involved in the transmission of bird song; many birds learn the form of their song from hearing other individuals sing. Dawkins (1976) has suggested the term 'meme' to cover culturally transmitted human ideas such as 'belief in life after death'.

Such learned behaviour is likely to be modified in the light of experience, and hence perhaps to be rather poorly transmitted over a long period of time, but in principle there is no reason why a culturally transmitted trait should not be subject to natural selection.

Behaviour genetics

Introduction

The study of the genetic basis of differences in behaviour is a flourishing field. A good introduction to the subject is given by McClearn and DeFries (1973), and a more advanced account by Ehrman and Parsons (1976). Where differences between species are being considered, the main effort has been devoted to a demonstration that the differences are hereditary. This can be done by rearing the species in the same environment and showing that the differences found in nature persist. For example, I have shown that if two species of titmice, the blue tit and the coal tit, are reared together in the laboratory, then many of the differences in feeding behaviour and habitat selection which are observed between the species in the wild are also observed in the laboratory. Further genetic analysis is usually impossible because in general different species will not hybridize even in the laboratory. Where differences in behaviour between members of the same species are being considered, the genetic analysis can be taken further by crossing individuals with particular phenotypes and observing the phenotypes of their progeny as described in the previous section.

Behaviour as a character for genetic analysis has several disadvantages. We have already noted that environmental influences acting on the phenotype can blur or mask genetic effects. This is especially pronounced for the behavioural phenotype, where learning can produce profound differences in behaviour between individuals or within one individual over time. Other changes in the internal state of animals can also affect their behaviour. For example, the level of circulating sex hormones in the body of a female mammal may vary with the stage of the oestrous cycle or the season of the year, and will produce dramatic differences in her behaviour from time to time. Hunger and thirst may also influence behaviour, not only towards food and water, but also in other contexts. In general it is fair to say that an animal's behaviour will be influenced by an enormous number of past and present environmental effects, and that therefore standardization of the conditions preceding and during measurement of behaviour are essential if the effects of genetic factors are to be successfully investigated. The behaviour of many animals including man varies with the time of day so that measurements should be carried out at the same time. Partly because of the many environmental effects on behaviour, most studies of behaviour genetics are concerned with continuously varying traits, although several major genes are known to affect behaviour.

Another problem for the study of behaviour genetics is that behaviour can be difficult to measure or categorize. Bodily movements are complicated three-dimensional occurrences with a particular temporal patterning. This problem is more acute in some cases than others; most people would agree on whether a chicken pecked or not in a certain time interval, but they might well disagree on whether two movements of a kitten during play were or were not the same. Accurate description and measurement are especially important in a study of behaviour because behavioural observations seem to be particularly prone to interference from subjective impressions and biases. In some cases the problem can be circumvented by the use of automatic recorders. Where this is not possible one simple procedure is to test whether a particular observer always classifies a particular behaviour in the same way. Another method of checking for consistency is to allow two independent observers to record their versions of the same sequence of events, and again to check for coincidence of their accounts. The problems of defining units of behaviour are taken up in Chapter 3.

Where groups of animals are being compared, one way of removing bias is to ensure that the experimenter does not know from which group the animal that he is testing has come. He cannot then produce spurious results by classifying borderline cases in accordance with his expectations.

Perhaps for these reasons much of the genetic analysis of behaviour has been concerned with fairly simple differences in behaviour which can be relatively easily measured.

Many mutants are likely to affect behaviour, because behaviour is the final expression of many processes going on in the animal. Because behaviour is produced by the nervous system, any mutant affecting the nervous system will affect behaviour. Many hormones affect behaviour, and any metabolic disorder is likely to impair the function of the nervous system. A change in external appearance may affect the behaviour of other individuals towards the affected individual, and hence may affect its own behaviour. There is no such thing as a purely behavioural mutant; the effect on behaviour must be mediated by processes occurring at other levels.

Major gene effects on behaviour

Although these effects are rare, there are examples in both animals and humans. One particularly elegant example is known in honeybees. In a beehive the queen lays an egg in each cell in the brood comb. These cells are then capped by the worker bees who feed the larvae and tend the brood comb. Occasionally these cells become infected by a bacterium which kills the larva, and if the larva is not removed and the cell cleaned the bacterial infection will spread to the rest of the colony. In most beehives the workers will uncap the affected cells and remove the infected larvae, and this has been called hygenic behaviour. Rothenbuhler (1964) has found that two independently transmitted genes on different chromosomes affect the two different aspects of this hygenic behaviour. By crossing the progeny of hygenic bees mated with bees from strains which do not show the hygenic behaviour, Rothenbuhler could produce hygenic individuals, individuals which would uncap cells but not remove dead larvae, individuals which would not uncap but which would remove dead larvae from cells which were already uncapped, and individuals which would neither uncap nor remove larvae.

Colour blindness in humans is produced by single alleles. There are a number of different forms of colour blindness, but the more common forms all have a similar genetic basis. To explain this, I will briefly describe how sex is determined in humans and other mammals. One of the 23 pairs of chromosomes in humans is involved in sex determination. Females have a pair of identical chromosomes, called X chromosomes, while males carry one X chromosome and a

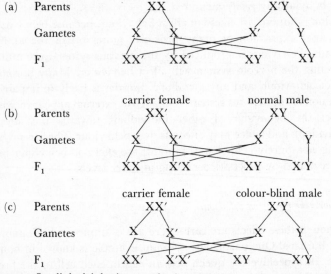

Fig. 1.3 Sex-linked inheritance of colour blindness in humans. (a) Cross between a colour-blind male and a normal female produces normal sons and carrier daughters. (b) Cross between a carrier female and a normal male produces daughters half of whom are normal and half carriers, and sons half of whom are normal and half colour-blind. (c) Cross between a carrier female and a colour-blind male produces daughters half of whom are carriers and half colour-blind and sons half of whom are normal and half colour-blind.

X = normal X chromosome, X′ = chromosome carrying allele for colour blindness, Y = Y chromosome.

differently shaped Y chromosome. Males produce gametes (spermatozoa) half of which contain an X chromosome, and half of which contain a Y. All female gametes (eggs) contain an X chromosome. Depending upon which of the two types of spermatozoa fertilize them, they produce a female (XX) or male (XY) individual. The point of this digression is that the mutation causing colour blindness is a recessive mutation carried on the X chromosome (a condition known as sex-linkage). The Y chromosome is genetically inert. Therefore if the mutation is present in a male it is expressed, while it has to be present in both X chromosomes in the female to be expressed. For this reason colour blindness is much more common in males than in females. The classic pattern of transmission is for an affected male to produce normal offspring, and for his daughters to produce sons half of whom are affected. This is explained in Figure 1.3.

Many mutant alleles whose presence is detected by biochemical means also affect behaviour. One example is the mutant causing phenylketonuria (PKU) in humans, which is associated with mental retardation. The disease results from an inability to metabolize the essential amino acid phenylalanine. The defect is caused by a recessive allele. It is now possible to screen babies both for the homozygous condition and for the heterozygous carrier condition. Individuals with the homozygous condition are given a diet which is low in phenylalanine, and may grow up to be normal in intelligence.

Chromosomal effects on complex behaviours and psychological processes

Chromosome imbalance can produce abnormalities in behaviour in animals and humans. The normal human chromosome complement is 23 pairs including the sex chromosomes. Individuals with Down's syndrome (mongolism) have 47 chromosomes, the extra one being a third copy of chromsome 21. These individuals have high infant mortality, and are usually severely mentally retarded. Sex chromosome abnormalities also occur in humans. Individuals with Klinefelter's syndrome are phenotypic males, but sexual development is abnormal, the affected individuals having abnormally small testes. They are sterile and many are mentally retarded. They are found to have one Y chromosome, and multiple X chromosomes, the most common form being XXY. Individuals with the sex chromosome complement XO (no Y chromosome and only one X) suffer from Turner's syndrome, and are sterile females. They also usually suffer from a defect in space perception.

Multiple gene effects on behaviour

Many behaviour traits have been found to be polygenically controlled. One such is geotaxis in the fruitfly. A selection experiment involving a T-maze in which the flies could either turn upwards (away from gravity) or downwards (towards gravity) showed a genetic basis to the behaviour, many genes being involved. Activity in mice, sexual behaviour in male rats and chickens, feeding behaviour in cattle and 'emotionality' in rats are all under polygenic control.

Several traits in man such as IQ, criminality and schizophrenia have been suggested to be under the control of many genes. The methodological problems associated with the study of human behaviour genetics are so enormous that the evidence for these claims should be treated with great caution. This is discussed in the next section.

Discussion

Genetics is concerned with the study of differences. If you were presented with a group of animals all of whom showed and bred true for a particular trait, such as green earlobes, you would not be able to determine the genetic basis of the trait. If the group contained a mixture of individuals with and without the trait then you could set about crossing individuals to examine the transmission of the trait to progeny. The fact that we are concerned with phenotypic differences when studying genetics leads to certain semantic problems, which especially where behaviour is concerned can lead to misconceptions.

We have seen that in the fruitfly differences in response to gravity (geotaxis) have some genetic basis. We cannot proceed from this discovery to a statement such as: 'Geotaxis is genetic', or 'Geotaxis is innate'. What we have shown is that some differences in geotactic behaviour are caused by genes. This does not mean that the environment plays no role in dictating the geotactic behaviour of a particular fly, or in bringing about differences in behaviour between flies. At the most obvious level inadequate nutrition may make the fly sluggish and unresponsive, but more adaptive modifications of behaviour in the light of experience may also be involved. To show that geotaxis was genetic, we would have to rule out the influence of environment in the development of the behaviour, and it is a truism that environment will *always* have some effect on behaviour, even if only to allow it to occur at all.

Another problem, particularly where behaviour is concerned, is that we have no idea what role genes play during development in producing the structure of the nervous system. Even if we could completely rule out environmental effects on behaviour, which we cannot, we could still not say with certainty that behaviour was genetic, because current ideas about development suggest that interactions between cells, and the position of cells in the body of an animal, may be important in determining what sort of structures they give rise to during development. The non-genetic part (the cytoplasm) of the gametes may be important in development, and again we could only detect its effects if individuals differed in respect of it.

Failure to make these distinctions has led to a rather pointless controversy between ethologists such as Lorenz, who emphasizes the evolutionary approach to behaviour, which of course has to be based on behaviour shown by nearly all members of a species (Lorenz calls such behaviour innate), and psychologists such as Lehrman, Hebb and Schneirla who have emphasized the role of learning and of environment in determining behaviour. Lehrman (1970) gives a clear account of the issues involved in this controversy.

Human behaviour genetics

As was mentioned in the previous section, differences in certain human traits such as intelligence, criminality and schizophrenia have been suggested to be under genetic control. It would be very surprising if many aspects of human behaviour and aptitudes did not have some genetic basis, but whether it is feasible to detect most genetic effects on human behaviour is doubtful because of the large environmental influences at work.

To separate the effects of heredity and environment, human genetics relies heavily on the use of family pedigrees, monozygotic (identical) twins reared together or in different environments, and adopted children of known parentage. The techniques have to be used because genticists cannot perform all the crosses that are necessary with humans, and because human environments cannot be manipulated or standardized. It is also extremely difficult to measure the relevant aspects of environment.

As this is a subject too large to be explored fully here, let us look at two examples of difficulties. Pedigrees of a particular trait such as schizophrenia are open to the criticism that close relatives are more likely to have similar environments than are more distant relatives. Therefore the demonstration of higher concordance for a trait between close relatives than between more distant ones could also be explained on the basis of similarities in environment.

Adoption studies would, at first sight, appear to provide the best means of partitioning differences between biological parentage and environment. This technique has been used, for example, in the study of the inheritance of IQ. Unfortunately, however, heredity and environment seem to go hand-in-hand in such studies for a reason which has only become apparent recently. This is that many adoption agencies try to match what they consider to be the characteristics of the adopting home with those of the home from which the child has come. This will produce a similarity in environment between the biological parents' home and the adopted parents' home, confounding any genetic influences which may be at work.

Probably the most convincing evidence is provided by studies of twins which compare monozygotic and dizygotic twins reared together and apart, but far more studies are needed.

It is particularly important with studies of human genetics that the results should be absolutely unambiguous before claims of genetic differences are made. This is because if such a claim were validated it would inevitably lead to discussion at a political level about matters such as educational policy, modification of the environment, and perhaps even eugenics. All of these would profoundly influence the lives of many human beings and so such discussion must be based on absolutely solid data. However, equal care needs to be taken regarding the kinds of conclusions that might be reached. For example, to suggest that because IQ might have some genetic basis it cannot therefore be modified or improved by education is tantamount to saying that because short-sight has a genetic basis sufferers should not be given glasses. The potential for incorrect and wrong-headed argument on these issues is enormous, whatever case is being presented. This is one of those areas of biology where the very greatest circumspection is required.

Social behaviour: individual selection, kin selection and game theory

In this section I shall assume that the social behaviour shown by animals has some heritable component and that it has evolved by the action of natural selection. Largely because of lack of study there is little evidence for a genetic basis to most social behaviour, but it is reasonable to assume that it has evolved in a similar way to other behaviour.

It is possible to understand many types of social behaviour in terms of evolution by conventional natural selection. Many birds such as starlings and pigeons feed in flocks, and it has been shown that at the approach of a predator one or more of the birds in the flock gives an alarm call in response to which all the birds fly away. In this situation one advantage of being in a flock is that on average some bird is likely to see the predator sooner than is a single bird feeding alone. In confirmation of this, small pigeon flocks in nature take evasive action at the approach of a predator later than do larger flocks, and as a consequence the predators have a higher success rate at catching a pigeon if they attack a small flock than if they attack a large one. Therefore it is of advantage to every member of the flock to participate in the group, because they all gain protection from predators, although there may be some loss of feeding efficiency because of competition for food with other flock members.

Many other examples of social behaviour can be understood in a similar way. Co-operative feeding such as group hunting by wolves and flock fishing by pelicans, and huddling for warmth in penguins can all be shown to benefit all the individuals involved, so that no special sort of mechanism need be invoked to understand their evolution.

It is less easy to understand some other forms of social behaviour as a product of individual selection. At first sight, parental care of the young by birds and mammals seems to need no special explanation. An individual's success under natural selection is measured by its number of surviving offspring, and any behaviour which increases this number will evolve. However, such an explanation is incomplete. The parental behaviour would not evolve unless the young also carried the genes causing them to show parental care in their turn. A parent which increases the chances of survival of its offspring by caring for them causes the genes for parental care to spread in the population because its offspring are both more numerous than the offspring of parents which do not care for their young, and because those more numerous young are likely to carry the gene causing them to show parental care. The interesting point here is that it is not only parents and offspring which have a heightened probability of carrying genes in common by descent. Siblings, first cousins, grandparents and their grandchildren all have a higher probability of carrying genes in common than do individuals taken at random from their population. Suppose that a mutation occurred which caused its bearer to help its siblings at some cost to itself, for example by sharing food. When the gene first arose it would be disadvantageous to its bearer because of the cost of food sharing. Because the mutation is new, the siblings of the bearer are highly unlikely to carry the mutation. If the bearer survives to breed, however, several of its offspring are likely to carry the food sharing gene. Though an offspring which shares food with its sibling will incur some cost to itself it will benefit its sibling who is also likely to carry the gene for food sharing. From this point on, whether the gene will spread in the population depends upon the cost to the 'altruist', the benefit to the recipient and the probability of the gene for food sharing being held in common. The act must increase the likelihood of survival of the mutation by more than the cost to the altruist reduces it. In general for the mutation to spread:

$$\text{benefit} > \frac{\text{cost}}{r}$$

where r = probability of holding the gene is common. It is higher for close relatives than for more distant ones.

This mechanism, which can explain the spread of apparently disadvantageous characters because of their beneficial effects on relatives, is called kin selection, and the behaviour so evolved is sometimes known as altruistic behaviour. Kin selection has been suggested as a mechanism for the evolution of the alarm calls mentioned earlier. The physical structure of these calls suggests that they have been subject to selection to make them hard to locate, presumably because they drew the attention of the predator to the caller. This suggests that they may have been disadvantageous to callers in comparison to non-

callers. However, the character could have evolved by kin selection
if the other members of the flock tend to be related to the caller.

Kin selection has also been invoked to explain the evolution of
sterile female worker bees who spend their lives looking after their
sisters, some of whom will be fertile queens. It is impossible to see how
sterility could evolve as a result of conventional individual selection.
Individual selection operates because certain organisms have higher
survival and reproductive success as a result of superiority of their
hereditary constitutions, and hence the particular alleles which caused
this superiority will increase in frequency in the next generation.
Sterility prevents an individual from transmitting its alleles to the next
generation, so that individual selection cannot act. In bees the males
are haploid, that is all their cells contain the number of chromosomes
present in the gametes. One consequence of this is that worker females
have a higher probability of holding genes in common with their
sisters than their own offspring (see Figure 1.4). A gene causing
a female to tend to her sisters at some cost to her own reproductive
effort might therefore spread, since one of her sisters will be the next

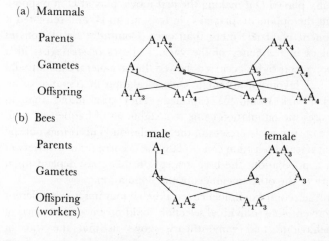

Fig. 1.4   The probability of sisters holding alleles in common. (a) In
mammals a cross between two parents with different alleles at the gene A
results in four classes of offspring, and the probability of two offspring
carrying a particular A allele in common is 50 per cent. (b) In bees,
because the males are haploid the offspring are certain to have the A allele
from their father in common, and have a 50 per cent probability of
carrying an A allele from their mother in common, so that the overall
probability of carrying a particular A allele in common is 75 per cent.

queen in the colony. For further discussion of social behaviour and kin selection see Dawkins (1976) and Wilson (1975).

The last topic to be considered is game theory, which has been used by Maynard Smith and Price (1973) to understand the evolution of behaviour in situations where the individuals involved have conflicting interests. This is particularly true of fights, where the winner may gain access to mates, dominance rights or a desirable territory, and where both contestants may run the risk of serious injury if the fighting becomes intense. In general most fights between animals do not result in serious injury.

Maynard Smith and Price considered various tactics which animals involved in fights might use, such as conventional (C) tactics which were unlikely to cause serious injury, and dangerous (D) tactics which were. They assigned scores to the possible outcomes of the fight. For example, in one of their fights they assigned a score of + 60 for winning, O for retreating uninjured, and − 100 for serious injury. Animals could play various combinations of D and C tactics. For example, one strategy called mouse never played D, while another called bully played D if making the first move, played D in response to C from the opponent, played C in response to D, and retreated if the opponent played D more than once. Computer simulations of the changes in frequency of the various classes of strategists in a population where fights occurred showed that in general conventional fighting was favoured, although some escalation in response to an escalated attack would be expected. They also found that in certain cases the population came to a stable set of frequencies with a mixture of strategists present in the population. This brings out the point that natural selection can explain the occurrence of a variety of forms in a population; the best strategy to take may depend upon the nature of the other members of the population.

Natural selection can influence social behaviour in several different ways. Conventional individual selection could produce many sorts of social behaviour, and game theory shows us that the way in which individual selection acts may depend upon the nature of the other individuals in the population. Kin selection can explain the evolution of traits which are disadvantageous to the individuals but have beneficial effects on relatives. There is one form of selection not yet mentioned which is called group selection. This mechanism of selection seeks to explain the evolution of individually disadvantageous characters on the basis of their beneficial effects on the group to which that individual belongs. For example, it has been suggested that groups composed of individuals who imposed upon themselves an individually disadvantageous limit to their reproduction would survive better than groups composed of selfish individuals who reproduced as much as possible and therefore depleted their food supply. A problem with group selection is that it relies upon the existence of isolated groups, because a selfish individual arriving in a group of altruists would breed faster than the altruists so that the group would come to be composed of selfish individuals. However, group selection may occur to some extent in nature. It is likely that all of these selective mechanisms have contributed to the evolution of social behaviour, and much work remains to be done to discover the contribution which each has made.

Note

1 I would like to thank Dr P. Ashmole for his helpful comments on the manuscript.

References

Cullen, E. (1957) Adaptations in the kittiwake to cliff-nesting. *Ibis 99*: 275–302.

Dawkins, R. (1976) *The Selfish Gene*. London: Oxford University Press.

Dobzhansky, T., Ayala, F. J., Stebbins, G. L. and Valentine, J. W. (1977) *Evolution*. San Francisco: W. H. Freeman.

Ehrman, L. and Parsons, P. A. (1976) *The Genetics of Behaviour*. Sunderland, Mass: Sinauer Associates Inc.

Koestler, A. (1971) *The Case of the Midwife Toad*. London: Pan Books.

Lehrman, D. S. (1970) Semantic and conceptual issues in the nature–nurture problem. In L. R. Aronson, E. Tobach, D. S. Lehrman and J. S. Rosenblatt, (eds) *Development and Evolution of Behaviour*. San Francisco: W. H. Freeman.

Maynard Smith, J. (1975) *The Theory of Evolution*. Third edn. Harmondsworth: Penguin Books.

Maynard Smith, J. and Price, G. R. (1973) The logic of animal conflict. *Nature 246*: 15–18.

McClearn, G. E. and DeFries, J. C. (1973) *Introduction to Behaviour Genetics*. San Francisco: W. H. Freeman.

Rothenbuhler, W. C. (1964) Behaviour genetics of nest cleaning in honeybees. IV. Responses of F_1 and backcross generations to disease-killed broods. *American Zoologist 4*: 111–23.

Srb, A. M., Owen, R. D. and Edgar, R. S. (1965) *General Genetics*. San Francisco: W. H. Freeman.

Wilson, E. O. (1975) *Sociobiology*. Belknap Press of Harvard University Press.

2 The anatomy of the vertebrate nervous system: an evolutionary and developmental perspective

Christopher H. Yeo

Introduction

The evolutionary history, or phylogeny, of modern-day vertebrates can be traced back to early, ancestral forms of some 500 million years ago. Diverse evolutionary paths from ancestral protochordates have led to the present vertebrate classes of fishes, amphibians, reptiles, birds and mammals (see Introduction to this volume, Figure 1). It may be shown that the changes which occurred during that enormous period of time which spans the animal's evolutionary history are to some extent recapitulated during its embryonic development from a fertilized egg to the adult form. The time-course of phylogeny is compressed many millionfold during the embryonic development, or ontogeny, of a modern vertebrate. This feature is nowhere more clearly seen than in the development of the nervous system and is of particular importance in the investigation of structure and function in this most complex of systems. There are surviving, contemporary species such as Amphioxus which have changed very little during phylogeny and so are very similar to the ancestral protochordates. The examination of the nervous systems of these, and of more advanced contemporary species, in the study of comparative neuroanatomy shows that there are fundamental similarities of structure and function in the nervous system of all vertebrates. Another consistent theme in the evolution of the vertebrate central nervous system is that newer structures and functions were super-imposed on existing ones rather than replacing them. Several examples of this process will be evident in the account which follows. For information on the evolution of the nervous system see Romer (1970, Chapter 16) and Sarnat and Netsky (1974). Comparative neuroanatomy is dealt with in the classic works of Papez (1929) and Kappers et al. (1936) and, more recently, in Pearson and Pearson (1976).

The basic elements

The fundamental unit of the nervous system is the electrically excitable nerve cell, or neuron. Like other living cells in the organism, the neuron has a cell body, or soma, which contains the nucleus and where the normal cellular metabolic processes occur. In addition, the soma bears a region of finely branching extensions, or dendrites, which serve to receive electrical information from other nerve cells and a single axon down which travels a wave of electrochemical output away from the soma. The axon may branch at one or several points to give axon collaterals.

In order to achieve a rapid conduction, the axons of vertebrate neurons may be sheathed in myelin, a fatty substance which acts as an electrical insulator. The myelin sheath is not continuous along the axon but has regularly spaced gaps – the nodes of Ranvier. These enable the characteristic 'jumping' or saltatory rapid conduction of the vertebrate myelinated nerve.

The most distal part of the axon is the terminal knob which abuts the next element in the neural circuit. Information is transmitted via specialized points of contact between the terminal knob of one neuron and a dendrite or perhaps the soma of the receiving neuron. These contact points are synapses, comprising a presynaptic and a postsynaptic element divided by a synaptic cleft about 0·02 microns wide. Whereas information is conducted as an electrochemical wave through the neuron, it crosses the synaptic cleft as brief pulses of a chemical neurotransmitter. The post-synaptic element receives the transmitter and the information content is recoded in the electrochemical form for further conduction.

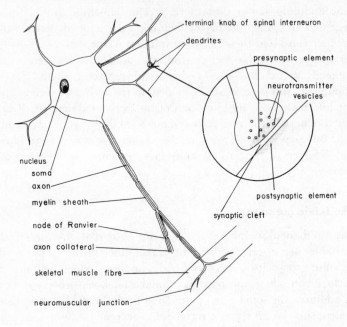

Fig. 2.1 Diagram of a spinal motoneuron, with input from an interneuron. The inset shows details of a synaptic connection.

For more detailed information on neurons and nerve action see Miles (1969) and Katz (1966).

In a neural circuit controlling muscle movement the final neuron in the sequence is known as a motoneuron. The special synaptic connection between motoneuron and muscle fibre is the neuromuscular junction. The neurotransmitter at the neuromuscular junctions of vertebrate skeletal muscle is acetylcholine (ACh). Other neurotransmitters found in the vertebrate nervous system include noradrenaline (also called norepinephrine), 5-hydroxytryptamine (5-HT or serotonin) and dopamine. A neurotransmitter with possible inhibitory action is gamma-amino-butyric acid (GABA) (see Chapter 4 of this volume).

Other neurons are specially adapted to react to non-neural events. These receptors are able to detect such stimuli as light, vibration or temperature and transduce such information to the electrochemical code of the nervous system. The receptors have axonal output to the next neuron in the circuit. Examples of such receptors are the rods and cones of the retina, hair cells in the cochlea of the ear and touch receptors in the skin.

Within the central nervous system (CNS), the cell bodies of neurons are often aggregated to form a nucleus, which should be distinguished from the intracellular structure of the same name. A similar aggregation in the peripheral nervous system is known as a ganglion. Axons, also, may be found collected in groups. An axon bundle in the CNS is known as a tract and in the peripheral nervous system as a nerve. Tracts which cross the midline are decussations. Decussating fibres which link similar areas on either side of the CNS are known as commissures.

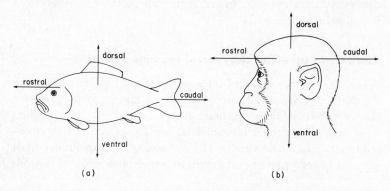

Fig. 2.2   The dorsal-ventral and rostral-caudal axes of (a) a fish – with horizontal body position, and (b) a primate – with upright stance.

Before the spatial configuration of the nervous system can be described, some commonly used terms should be defined. The locations of structures within the brain are usually described with reference to the dorsal-ventral and the rostral-caudal axes (see Figures 2.2a and b). These terms are unambiguous for animals with horizontal bodies but they may be confused when describing positions in the primate brain, since the body is upright in these animals. The ambiguity is resolved by considering monkeys, apes and men as 'horizontal' animals with a head position distorted backwards through 90°. The axes are then as shown in Figure 2.2b with the top of the head being dorsal and so on. From early stages of embryonic development the vertebrate brain is predominantly bilaterally symmetrical (see Chapter 8 of this volume). With the exception of structures such as the cerebellum on the midline, the components on the CNS are duplicated – one on the left and one on the right side. Thus the location of a structure may be completely described in terms of the rostral-caudal and dorsal-ventral axes and whether it is medial (close to the midline) or lateral (to the right or left side). When two structures appear on the same side of the CNS they are said to be ipsilateral and, conversely, if on opposite sides they are contralateral.

Two terms which have functional rather than anatomical significance are afferent and efferent. An afferent neuron conveys information towards a particular centre (for example, a touch receptor in the skin is afferent to the spinal cord) whereas an efferent neuron conveys information away from a centre (for example, a motoneuron is a spinal cord efferent).

The neural tube and the central nervous system

A vertebrate nervous system of the very simplest type may be seen in the early embryos of advanced vertebrates and in adult, primitive chordates. It is of a tubular shape, formed by an infolding or invagination of the dorsal ectoderm (see Figure 2.3). This segmented neural tube is a nerve network surrounding a central lumen. Each segment bears a pair of dorsal, sensory nerves and a pair of ventral,

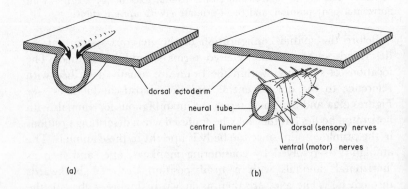

Fig. 2.3   The development of the neural tube from dorsal ectoderm. In (a) the ectoderm has begun to invaginate; in (b) the neural tube has differentiated, and segmental nerves have developed.

motor nerves. In this primitive state, intrasegmental connections between sensory and motor elements allow only a very ,limited behavioural repertoire confined to very simple reflexive acts. In order that complex behaviours may be organized, intersegmental connections have developed and the rostral part of the neural tube has become the brain – a centre of higher control in more evolved forms (see Figure 2.4a). This process of encephalization has occurred to different degrees and with various eleborations in the brains of the five vertebrate classes (see Figure 2.5; see also Chapters 6 and 7 of this volume). Consistent with the brain's operation as a control centre is the input of information from the so-called 'distance' receptors. Visual, auditory and olfactory inputs converge directly upon the brain, enabling response decisions to be made centrally, and in advance of contact with the object or event which is giving rise to the stimulus. The output of the system also becomes improved by the development of direct motor connections from the brain to the segments of the neural tube and thence to the muscles. At this stage of development the neural tube may be seen as consisting of two parts – the brain and the spinal cord. The embryonic origins are recognized in the consideration of the brain and the spinal cord as a single functional unit – the central nervous system.

The peripheral nervous system

In its role as a central integrator of information, the CNS requires inputs to supply it with information about its surroundings and outputs to deliver its instructions to the effectors – the muscles and glands. These functions are fulfilled by the peripheral nervous system (PNS), which in man consists of 31 pairs of spinal nerves which, as their name implies, enter the spinal cord, and 12 pairs of cranial nerves which enter the brain directly.

The PNS comprises somatic and visceral components. Somatic motor fibres innervate skeletal muscles enabling voluntary movements, and somatic sensory fibres are from the exteroceptive receptors for stimuli such as touch and heat. The cell bodies of somatic sensory neurons lie in the two chains of dorsal root ganglia – one chain on each side of the spinal cord. Visceral sensory fibres are from the interoceptive receptors such as stretch receptors in the gut, and visceral motor fibres innervate smooth muscle and glands. Because of its seemingly self-governing nature in controlling the internal environment of the animal, the visceral efferent component is usually referred to as the autonomic system (ANS).

The ANS of most vertebrates comprises two subsystems which each innervate a particular organ but have contrasting actions. Fibres of the sympathetic system are found in the spinal nerves of thoracic (chest region) and lumbar (back region) segments, while those of the parasympathetic system are in the sacral (tail region) spinal nerves and in some cranial nerves, particularly the vagus. Activity in the sympathetic system causes, amongst other effects, increases in heart and respiratory rates and slowing down of digestive processes. Parasympathetic activity causes the reverse of these effects. Apart from the anatomical differences, the neurotransmitters of the sympathetic and parasympathetic systems are different. Noradrenaline is the neurotransmitter of the sympathetic system whereas acetylcholine is found in the parasympathetic system.

The sympathetic–parasympathetic double innervation of organs is not completely developed in the earliest evolved vertebrates. Where this is the case, control is either by the sympathetic or by the parasympathetic system alone. The heart of the teleost fish, for instance, is innervated only by the vagus, which maintains control by exerting tonic, inhibitory influence over the intrinsically rapid heart rate.

The development of the brain

In order to describe the general form of the vertebrate brain, let us now consider the embryonic development of the generalized brain indicated in Figure 2.4. In the first stage (Figure 2.4a), the most rostral part of the embryonic neural tube develops three swellings, later to become the hindbrain, the midbrain and the forebrain. At the second stage (Figure 2.4b), the forebrain is seen to have divided into the telencephalon and the diencephalon (the thalamus and hypothalamus); the olfactory bulbs become differentiated. In the hindbrain, the cerebellum, pons and medulla may be distinguished. The dorsal part of the midbrain develops the superior and inferior colliculi. Stage three (Figure 2.4c) only occurs to completion in the mammal, where there is considerable development of the telencephalon, ultimately to form the cerebral hemispheres. The telencephalon bulges outwards and evaginates, folding back over the brainstem in order to accommodate itself within the confines of the

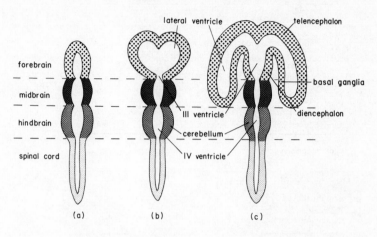

Fig. 2.4   The development of the brain and spinal cord from the neural tube (the spinal cord is shown shortened for convenience). Spinal cord, hindbrain, midbrain and forebrain are shown stippled as indicated. The central lumen is shown as an unstippled area.

skull. The older parts of the telencephalon which become enfolded between the outermost cortical layer and the thalamus are the archicortex, and the striatum or basal ganglia. The most recently developed part of the telencephalon is the neopallium, more usually called neocortex. This mantle of folded neural tissue reaches its greatest level of development in man, where its massive, fissured structure enables the maximum surface area of cortex to be achieved. Figure 2.5 shows the brains of representatives of the vertebrate classes. The trend towards increased telencephalic development in the mammal is clearly shown.

In summary, during both ontogenetic and phylogenetic development the neural tube becomes progressively differentiated by the process of encephalization. Initially, separate brain and spinal cord regions are formed, and subsequently there is elaboration and expansion of the brain itself, particularly its rostral components (see Chapter 6 of this volume). In the Introduction to this book, the traditional description of birds and mammals as 'higher' vertebrates and fishes, amphibians and reptiles as 'lower' vertebrates has been discussed. As all of these vertebrate types have successful living representatives, the unqualified terms of 'higher' and 'lower' vertebrates with their evaluative overtones are potentially mis-

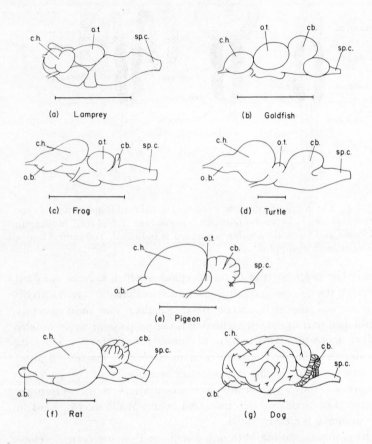

Fig. 2.5 Lateral views of the external features of seven vertebrate brains representing: (a) a cyclostome fish; (b) a teleost fish; (c) an amphibian; (d) a reptile; (e) a bird; (f) a mammal with non-convoluted cerebral hemispheres (= lissencephalic); (g) a mammal with convoluted cerebral hemispheres (= gyrencephalic) (see also the Introduction to this volume, especially Figure 1). Below each brain, and on the same individual scale, the calibration bar represents 1 cm.

Abbreviations: cb. = çerebellum; c.h. = cerebral hemisphere; o.b. = olfactory bulb; o.t. = optic tectum; sp.c. = spinal cord.

leading. Within the evolutionary perspective of this chapter, birds and mammals will be described as more encephalized, and fishes, amphibians and reptiles are less encephalized vertebrates.

The lumen of the neural tube has also been affected by the process of CNS differentiation to form the ventricles of the brain and the central canal of the spinal cord. As a result of their common origin the central canal of the spinal cord is continuous with the ventricular system of the brain, and both contain cerebrospinal fluid (CSF). The central canal connects with the fourth ventricle of the hindbrain, which in turn connects with the more rostral third ventricle via the narrow Aqueduct of Sylvius in the midbrain. The largely diencephalic third ventricle gives off two lateral ventricles inside the cerebral hemispheres (see Figure 2.4c).

The entire brain and spinal cord are enclosed in a series of three membranes or meninges. The outermost covering is the tough, protective dura mater. Immediately beneath this is the delicate, spongy arachnoid mater which sends spidery projections to the innermost membrane, the pia mater. The space between the arachnoid and the pia mater, the subarachnoid space, is filled with CSF. Blood vessels in the arachnoid mater and subarachnoid space send branches through the pia mater to supply oxygen and other nutrients to the surface of the brain.

The general organization of a vertebrate brain as seen in vertical section is shown schematically in Figure 2.6. At this point, it is useful to consider the detailed anatomy of the CNS, starting by

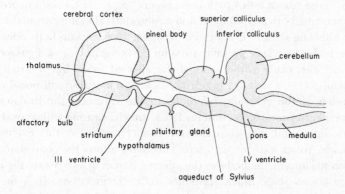

Fig. 2.6   A vertical section through a generalized vertebrate brain.

looking at the spinal cord. This is the least changed part of the neural tube, and shows features of the more developed brain regions.

The spinal cord

Since the spinal cord retains many of the features of the simple neural tube, it is structurally rather similar in the different vertebrate classes. Ascending and descending tracts, supplying the brain with sensory information and carrying its integrated output to the peripheral nervous system, form a large part of the spinal cord but it also has considerable autonomy in the control of the simple behavioural sequences known as reflexes. Figure 2.7 shows transverse sections of the spinal cord. Immediately recognizable are an outer region of white matter, composed of the myelinated fibres of ascending and descending tracts, and a central region of grey matter, comprising cell bodies and small, unmyelinated fibres.

Reflexes are organized in the spinal cord by relatively few connections between sensory and motor neurons. Figure 2.7a shows some examples of these reflex arcs. Input from the receptor passes down the sensory nerve fibre, past the cell body in the dorsal root ganglion, and enters the cord by the dorsal horn of the central grey matter. Here the fibre may give off axon collaterals to higher or lower segments of the cord. Connections to motoneurons in the same segment are shown in the diagram. In most instances, connections to the motoneuron involve a short interneuron in the grey matter; this is a disynaptic pathway. Figure 2.7a shows interneurons connecting both an ipsilateral and a contralateral motoneuron, thereby allowing sensory input to influence motor events on both sides of the body. A relatively mild stimulus to the skin (e.g. a light pin-prick) can cause withdrawal of the affected limb, but a stronger stimulus (e.g. a stronger pin-prick, a burn) may cause additional extension of the contralateral limb. In this instance, the ipsilateral motoneuron connection is to the flexor muscle, causing withdrawal of the limb, and the contralateral connection is to the extensor muscle, which extends the limb. This reflex allows the contralateral limb to support the body as the affected part is drawn away. Figure 2.7a shows some much simplified reflex connections. It is more usual that many motoneurons are influenced by a sensory input, either by connections derived from the sensory axon collaterals

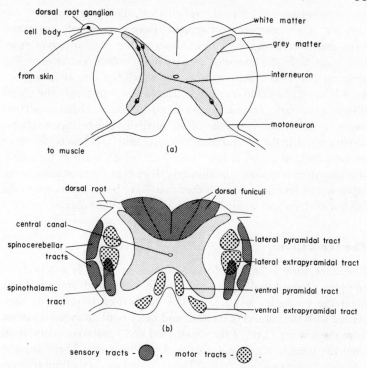

Fig. 2.7   Diagrams of transverse sections through the spinal cord showing (a) reflex arcs and (b) tracts.

shown ascending and descending in the dorsal horn, or by other projections from the interneuron.

The major tracts of the spinal cord are shown in Figure 2.7b. The sensory pathways include the dorsal funiculi, which project to the medulla. The spinocerebellar tract projects to the cerebellum and the lateral and ventral spinothalamic tracts terminate in the thalamus. The motor pathways from the brain include the extrapyramidal tracts from the subcortical motor areas, and the ventral pyramidal tract from the motor cortex. The lateral pyramidal tract consists of decussated fibres from the motor cortex.

The medulla and pons

The hindmost part of the brain is the medulla, which retains a structure rather similar to the spinal cord. The grey matter of the medulla has, however, dissociated from its spinal, columnar form and is arranged as nuclei. Many of the cranial nerves enter and leave from the medulla and its more rostral extension – the pons; in particular, the vagus nerve which, as has already been described, controls vital respiratory and cardiac functions. The nuclei of these important nerves are located in the medulla. Other important nuclei in this region are those of the medially placed raphé system, which are rich in the neurotransmitter serotonin (5-HT), and the more laterally located nuclei of locus coeruleus, which serve as the origin of major noradrenaline containing pathways in the brain. Both the raphé nuclei and those of locus coeruleus have been implicated in the control of sleep and waking (see Chapter 5 of this volume).

The cerebellum

The cerebellum is located dorsally above the pons. It is a body of complex, convoluted appearance, with a fissured cortical layer overlying its nuclei and tracts. The cerebellum is primarily concerned with the control of balance and movement and receives input from the sensory fibres of the spinal cord and vestibular information from the semicircular canal system of the inner ear. There are also auditory and visual projections. The mammalian cerebellum receives considerable cortical input through the pons. The output of the cerebellum is via separate cerebellar nuclei to the ventrolateral thalamus and onwards to the motor cortex and the pyramidal tract. Other outputs are to the vestibular nuclei and the extrapyramidal motor system.

The midbrain

The midbrain is clearly divisible into dorsal and ventral regions. The dorsal part bears two paired bodies – the superior and inferior colliculi. The former are important visual nuclei, and the latter receive auditory connections. In fish and amphibians the superior colliculus, or optic tectum, is the most important visual centre. The fibres of the optic tract enter the brain at the thalamus, but most pass on to terminate in a precise topographic manner on the surface of the optic tectum, forming a 'map' of the visual world in the brain. Auditory, vestibular and somatosensory information also projects here, and motor information is delivered to the effectors via the tectospinal tract. In fish and amphibians the tectum is the most important correlative centre of the brain, but in birds and mammals the forebrain has developed to dominate this phylogenetically older structure.

The ventral part of the midbrain is known as the tegmentum. This is a felt-like mass of cell bodies and interconnecting nerve fibres, and is the central part of the reticular formation, a diffuse system which extends through the brainstem from the medulla to the thalamus. The brain stem reticular formation has an ascending component which projects to the thalamus and the cerebral cortex. It functions to 'alert' the cortex when sensory input is arriving, and mediates the arousal response which may be detected by recording an electroencephalogram. The reticular formation also has a descending component which influences activity in the extrapyramidal motor system. Also in the tegmentum are the red nucleus and substantia nigra, both of which are parts of the extrapyramidal motor system. Substantia nigra is the origin of an important dopamine containing pathway, the nigrostriatal bundle, which projects to the striatum.

The thalamus and epithalamus

The thalamus is situated in the diencephalon, just rostral to the mid-brain, and is a bilateral aggregation of many different nuclei. A useful description of the thalamus divides these nuclear groups into three different categories: sensory relay nuclei, association nuclei and intrinsic nuclei.

Sensory relay nuclei receive direct input from ascending sensory fibres and project forward to sensory regions of the forebrain. In fish and amphibians, the thalamus receives mainly visual information, but this is over-shadowed by projections from other sensory systems in the mammal. The lateral geniculate nucleus receives retinal fibres and projects forward to visual cortex in the mammal and to the striatum in the bird. In less encephalized vertebrates the forebrain projections appear to be rather less specific, and it seems likely that the teleost fish has no telencephalic visual projection at all.

Association nuclei of the thalamus receive non-direct sensory information and have projections to association areas of the forebrain. An association nucleus of the visual system is the nucleus rotundus or pulvinar. This nucleus receives input from the optic tectum and has connections to visual association cortex.

Intrinsic nuclei may be considered to be a continuation of the midbrain reticular formation. Stimulation of these nuclei causes wide-spread activation of most cortical areas, and they are therefore considered to be components of a diffuse thalamic activating system. Apart from these important connections with the reticular formation, the intrinsic nuclei of the thalamus have connections with the limbic system.

The dorsal diencephalon is known as the epithalamus, which comprises the habenula and the pineal gland. The habenulae are paired structures with important connections to the olfactory system, and are markedly asymmetrical in most animals. It has been suggested that the habenula regulates feeding behaviour in less encephalized forms and newly born mammals

The hypothalamus

The hypothalamus is another major diencephalic structure and lies ventral to the thalamus, as its name suggests. The nuclei of the hypothalamus are highly involved in the regulation of eating, drinking and sexual behaviours. In association with other elements of the limbic system it is also concerned in the regulation of emotional behaviour. The hypothalamus exerts control over the underlying pituitary gland – the master endocrine gland. By this means, the hypothalamus is able to control many of the endocrine functions of the body, including the regulation of ovulation in the female and levels of thyroid activity.

The telencephalon

The telencephalon, or cerebrum, is formed from paired swellings of the rostral end of the neural tube (see Figures 2.4b and c), and it shows greater variations of structure within the vertebrate classes than any other region of the brain.

Three main divisions of the telencephalon may be recognized: the paleocortex, which is a phylogenetically old structure, seen as the pyriform lobes; the archicortex, which is represented by the hippocampus and the septum; and the neocortex, which appears first in reptiles and develops greatly in mammals. In addition the oldest parts of the neocortex, the cingulate cortex and entorhinal cortex, are sometimes classed separately as intermediate cortex. A fourth region, which is not described as cortical, consists of the basal ganglia. This group of nuclei (they are not true ganglia) originated in the walls of the telecephalon but are found centrally within the cerebral hemispheres in species in which there is advanced neocortical development. The basal ganglia consist of the corpus stria-

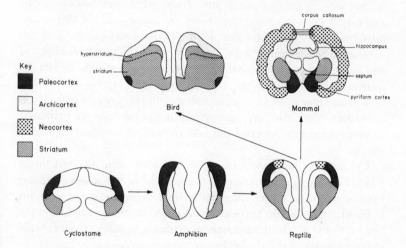

Fig. 2.8 Diagrams of transverse sections through the forebrains of five vertebrates. Paleo-, archi- and neocortex and striatum are indicated as shown in the key, and ventricular space is shown unshaded. Based on Sarnat and Netsky (1974).

tum (caudate nucleus, putamen and globus pallidus) and the amygdala. Strictly, the term cerebral cortex includes all telencephalic cortical regions, but it is commonly used to describe neocortex only.

Figure 2.8 shows transverse sections through the forebrains of five vertebrate types. Cyclostome (jawless fish) and amphibian forebrains have small cerebral lobes of archi- and paleocortex. The reptilian forebrain is rather similar, but has a more developed striatum, and neocortex has emerged dorsally. The avian forebrain shows massive development of the striatum (also see Figure 2.5) which becomes the most important integrative region in birds. It may be divided into the ectostriatum and an additionally developed part, the hyperstriatum, or Wulst.

The mammalian forebrain is characterized by large neocortical expansion, and in some mammals this neocortical area is further increased by fissuring of the surface (see Figure 2.5). The basal ganglia come to occupy a central position within the hemispheres and direct striatal-neocortical connections are established. The archicortical hippocampus and septum are easily distinguishable.

The mammalian telencephalon has developed interhemispheric connections via the corpus callosum. It seems that information may be exchanged between the hemispheres by means of this huge commissure, the largest fibre tract in the brain (see Chapter 8 of this volume). The corpus callosum can be subdivided on both anatomical and functional grounds into the genu rostrally, a central body and the splenium caudally. Other commissures are represented in all vertebrate classes: the anterior commissure interconnects archicortical structures, and also the neocortical temporal lobe in primates. Commissures of the superior and inferior colliculi are also found in all species.

The mammalian neocortex comprises three particular functional types. Sensory cortex receives projections from the sensory systems via thalamic relay nuclei. Information from particular sensory systems is directed to specific cortical regions, which all lie caudal to the central fissure of advanced mammalian brains. Somatic sensory cortex is immediately behind the fissure, auditory cortex is lateral, in the temporal lobe, and visual cortex is near the back of the brain in

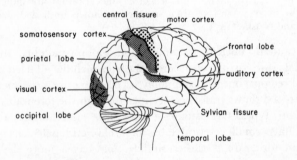

Fig. 2.9 The cerebral cortex of man, showing the four lobes, the major fissures, and sensory and motor cortex. Untoned areas are association cortex.

the occipital poles. The projection of information onto sensory cortex is in a precise, orderly manner. This is clearly seen in the projection of somatosensory information from the receptors in the skin (see Figure 2.10a).

A very similar orderly arrangement is seen in the region of motor cortex which lies just rostral to the central fissure (see Figure 2.10b). Motor cortex gives projections to the pyramidal and extra-pyramidal motor systems.

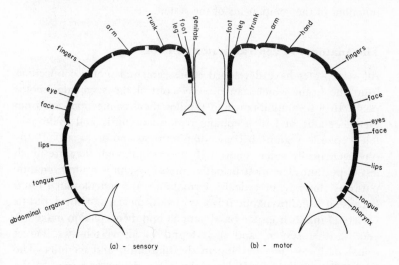

Fig. 2.10   Topographical representations of (a) somatosensory cortex and (b) motor cortex in man. Notice the increased representation for dextrous and sensitive regions, such as fingers and lips.

A third type of cortex, sometimes termed association cortex, has neither direct sensory input nor motor inputs. The proportion of this type of cortex increases markedly in the primates, culminating in very large association areas, which include the frontal lobes in man. Association cortex is classified as 'silent' in those regions which are not responsive to peripheral stimuli whilst other areas which are activated indirectly by all varieties of stimuli are described as polysensory.

In the preceding description of the structure of the telencephalon, the various components of the limbic system have been described individually but, because of the significance of the interconnection of these components, they should also be considered as a system. The limbic system in mammals forms a border (= limbus) around the junction between the thalamus and the medial surface of the cerebral hemisphere and includes the hippocampus, the amygdala, the septum, pyriform cortex and cingulate cortex. These structures are strongly interconnected, and also have hypothalamic associations. Lesions of the limbic system produce a variety of disturbances of emotional behaviour, but there remains much doubt about the individual functions of the components of the system.

The anatomy of central motor control

All vertebrates have developed suprasegmental motor connections from the brain which can directly control the segmental motor pools. In fish, amphibians and reptiles these connections are from mesencephalic and diencephalic regions; in birds and mammals, telencephalic regions become dominant as motor areas but the phylogenetically older connections persist, although they are much less important. The most primitive motor system is a multisynaptic pathway through the reticular formation – the reticulospinal tract. Because it is multisynaptic it is a very slow means of control, but its variety of inputs from the basal ganglia and diencephalon make it a very flexible system, and it is found in all vertebrates. Direct spinal pathways first develop in the hindbrain and medulla. The medial longitudinal fasciculus is the oldest descending tract in the CNS and carries information from the vestibular nuclei and the cerebellum to the spinal cord. As the principal centre of coordination in the lower vertebrate brain, the optic tectum exerts direct motor control via the tectospinal tract. In more encephalized vertebrates vestibular information remains an important spinal input, via the lateral vestibulospinal tract. The reticulospinal tract is still to be found, but it has developed a direct connection, by-passing the old multisynaptic pathway.

The development of the forebrain allows a shifting of motor control into these higher regions. The extrapyramidal motor system becomes developed in recently evolved vertebrates and is centred around the basal ganglia, particularly the striatum. The connections of the system are complex and the description which follows is much simplified. The caudate nucleus and putamen have inputs to the globus pallidus (all of these are striatal structures) which in turn feeds its output to the subthalamic and other brainstem nuclei such as the red nucleus of the tegmentum. From these, the motor commands descend via the ipsilateral and contralateral extrapyramidal tracts. The striatum receives important ascending influences from the substantia nigra via the dopaminergic nigrostriatal bundle. In the mammal, the basal ganglia have many reciprocal connections with most areas of the neocortex, including motor and sensory cortex. These connections are important in the mammalian extrapyramidal system – it seems that cortical information is used in motor control by this system, but it is likely that the basal ganglia are dominant.

Mammals have developed another direct system of motor control which is known as the pyramidal motor system (because it passes through the medullary pyramids – large triangular swellings on the base of the medulla). This system is a direct connection between neurons of the motor cortex (see Figures 2.9 and 2.10b) and spinal motoneurons. It is this system which allows the representation of the body musculature along the cortical motor strip. The fibres descend through the brainstem and many decussate in the caudal medulla. The ipsilateral component passes through the ventral corticospinal tract; the decussated component is the lateral corticospinal tract. It would appear that the pyramidal tract is most important in primates and man, since lesions of this system produce only transient deficits in other mammals whereas in primates very long-lasting or permanent deficits in fine, skilled movements may be seen.

The anatomy of central sensory systems – vision

The increasing importance of the forebrain through the phylogenetic series is not restricted to its motor control functions; in sensory systems, too, the role of the telencephalon increases in more encephalized vertebrates. This evolutionary trend is well illustrated in the development of the visual system. The structure of the retina is fairly constant throughout the vertebrates. Light is detected by the receptors in the innermost layer of the retina, at the back of the eye. These receptors synapse upon retinal bipolar cells which, in turn, synapse upon the retinal ganglion cells (see Figure 2.11). The ganglion cells have long axons, which lead out from the back of the eye as the optic nerve.

There are two regions of lateral interconnections in the retina; first, a layer of horizontal cells immediately below the receptors and,

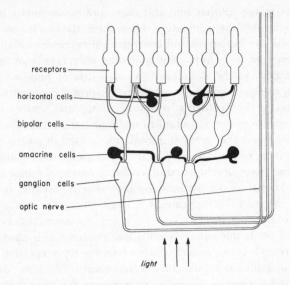

receptors ──────

horizontal cells──────

bipolar cells ──────

amacrine cells──────

ganglion cells ──────

optic nerve ──────

light

Fig. 2.11   A diagrammatic representation of a transverse section through a vertebrate retina. Note that light travels through the neural tissue to the receptors at the back of the retina. The ganglion cell fibres traverse the surface of the retina, and pierce it centrally, to run back to the brain as the optic nerve.

second, a layer of amacrine cells at the junction of the bipolar and ganglion cells. Connections between these components allow a certain amount of processing of visual information within the retina, before it is supplied to the brain (Michael, 1969).

It should be noted that light impinging on the retina must travel through the ganglion and bipolar cell layer before reaching the receptors. This curious arrangement may be due to the evolution of the eye from photosensitive tissue on the surface of the primitive dorsal ectoderm. With the invagination of both of these tissues in the formation of the neural tube, the photosensitive region came to lie within the neural tube. The tube then proceeded to 'bud off' a pair of optic vesicles which later become the eye. The position of the photoreceptors remained constant, below the overlying neural tissue. This resulted in the 'inverted' arrangement of the retinal receptor layer (for a full account of this theory, see Sarnat and Netsky, 1974, Chapter 8).

In non-mammalian vertebrates the optic nerves are completely decussated, i.e. each optic nerve terminates in the contralateral side of the brain. The optic nerves cross over (decussate) at the optic chiasm, from where they proceed to enter the brain as the optic tracts (strictly, the entire optic nerve is a tract since the retina should be regarded as part of the brain itself). Decussation at the chiasm is not complete in most mammals. In the rat, 10 per cent of the optic nerve fibres pass to the ipsilateral side of the brain. This figure rises to 50 per cent in primates. Ipsilateral fibres arise from the temporal region of the retina which receives input from the nasal (central) part of the visual field.

In the fish, the majority of optic nerve fibres synapse on the contralateral optic tectum. A very small component terminates on various nuclei of the dorsal thalamus, but in teleost fish there is no projection to the forebrain (see Figure 2.12).

In the bird, the retinotectal projection remains, but the tectum relays its visual input to the nucleus rotundus, which then projects forward to the ectostriatum of the telencephalon. In addition to this phylogenetically older system a second pathway has developed. Some of the optic nerve fibres terminate in the geniculate nucleus of the thalamus and this relays a projection to the massively developed hyperstriatum, or Wulst. Thus, in the bird, the striatum is the important sensory forebrain region, with neocortical development remaining slight.

In the mammal, a retino-geniculate-neocortical pathway has become the dominant visual pathway. Retinal fibres synapse at the lateral geniculate nucleus of the thalamus and are relayed to the visual cortex at the occipital lobe of the cortex (Hubel, 1963). This primary visual cortex also relays information to the surrounding visual association cortex. Although this central visual pathway is of prime importance in the mammal, the retinotectal pathway is also still present. A small proportion of retinal fibres terminate on the superior colliculus, which is the mammalian homologue of the optic tectum of lower vertebrates. The superior colliculus has projections to the pulvinar (= nucleus rotundus) which itself has ascending connections to visual association cortex. It seems that, in the absence of the cortical system, the collicular pathway can still subserve visual functions. Animals with extensive lesions of the visual cortex retain considerable visual ability and it is suggested that this is mediated by the collicular pathway (see Chapters 7 and 8 of this volume).

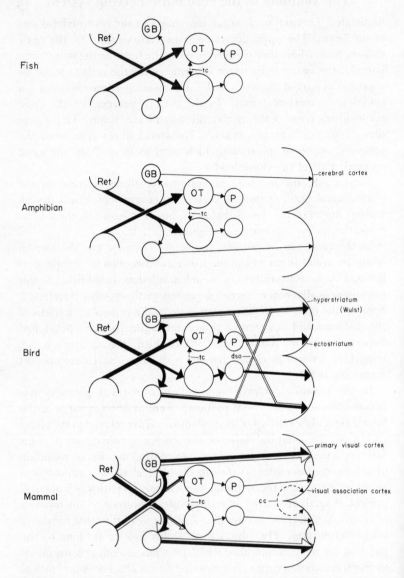

Fig. 2.12 The major visual pathways in four types of vertebrate. Abbreviations: dso = supraoptic decussation; cc = corpus callosum; GB = geniculate body; OT = optic tectum; P = pulvinar; Ret = retina; tc = tectal commissure. The pulvinar is usually known as the nucleus rotundus in non-mammalian forms, and the mammalian optic tectum is also known as the superior colliculus.

Conclusions

In the preceding pages the reader has been introduced to the investigation of the anatomy of the nervous system from ontogentic and phylogenetic viewpoints. It can be seen that the complexities of the nervous systems of the more encephalized animals are superimposed on older, simpler systems. There seems little doubt that this hierarchical arrangement of central control enables the unique flexibilities of behaviour which are the property of the highest vertebrates, reaching their present peak of development in the central nervous system of man.

References

Hubel, D. H. (1963) The visual cortex of the brain. *Scientific American 209*: 54–62.

Kappers, C. U. A., Huber, G. C. and Crosby, E. C. (1936) *The Comparative Anatomy of the Nervous System of Vertebrates, Including Man*. New York: Macmillan (reprinted by Hafner, New York, 1960).

Katz, B. (1966) *Nerve, Muscle and Synapse*. New York: McGraw-Hill.

Michael, C. R. (1969) Retinal processing of visual images. *Scientific American 220*: 104–14.

Miles, F. A. (1969) *Excitable Cells*. London: Heinemann.

Papez, J. W. (1929) *Comparative Neurology*. New York: Hafner.

Pearson, R. and Pearson, L. (1976) *The Vertebrate Brain*. London: Academic Press.

Romer, A. S. (1970) *The Vertebrate Body*. Philadelphia: Saunders.

Sarnat, H. B. and Netsky, M. G. (1974) *Evolution of the Nervous System*. New York: Oxford University Press.

3 Brain-behaviour studies and evolutionary biology[1]

H. C. Plotkin

Introduction

The attempt to understand and relate central nervous system structure and function to behaviour has assumed major importance to the neurosciences in general and to psychology in particular. Physiological psychology (or behavioural physiology, as some prefer) is a very old subject – conceptually at least as old as Descartes. As an experimental science it has been in existence for over 100 years. Yet it is very largely a twentieth-century achievement, and even more so one of the last two decades. This recent burgeoning of activity is directly related to the massive surge of output from the neurosciences at large. Refined techniques of lesion induction, degeneration studies, aggregate and unit recording and analysis of cellular activity, and neurochemical and neuropharmacological analyses have been gradually drafted into brain-behaviour studies. At the same time the neurosciences have begun to accept the value of behavioural data as a functional expression of brain activity. Thus, for example, visual discrimination learning in rats with lesions of the visual system is now considered as valid a form of study of the neurological substrata of vision as, say, the determination of the receptive fields of cells in striate cortex. A logical progression from such thinking has been the use of behaviour as a measure of brain manipulation, and indeed the field produces its strongest data when both physiological and behavioural measures agree in such studies. For example, if kittens are reared under conditions of restricted visual experience then their visual systems will show a lack of physiological sensitivity to lines of orientation which corresponds to the early visual deprivation. They are also behaviourally blind, the blindness again corresponding to the form of visual deprivation suffered by the animals during development. The net outcome of this increase in new techniques together with the growth in the use of behaviour by neuroscientists has been an explosion in the number of brain-behaviour studies being carried out and reported.

Evolutionary psychobiology, the attempt to understand behaviour within the context of evolutionary biology, also has a long history – and a distinguished one in so far as it begins with Darwin himself. However, the continuity of this approach has been poor and but for the European ethologists, who quite specifically advocated evolution as the central tenet around which to build a science of behaviour, it might not have survived. But keep it alive they did, and more than that, their influence on recent behavioural science has ranged widely from learning theory (Seligman and Hager, 1972, for example) through to social behaviour (Wilson, 1975). Mason and Lott (1976) suggest that the reason for this recent upsurge of interest in the evolution of behaviour lies in the realization that behaviour is a 'major evolutionary achievement' and 'a fundamental activity of the organism as a whole play(ing) a central role in day-to-day adjustments'. The relationship between behaviour and evolution is no simple matter, and the logic, which is complex and subtle, has yet to be properly worked out. The problem, briefly, is that unlike most other phenotypic traits, behaviour is 'active' and simultaneously occupies a dual position in the evolutionary process. This is because behaviour is at once the product of evolution (just as is any other phenotypic character) and yet at the same time is one of the major determinants of the selection pressures acting upon an animal, in that it is one of the most important means by which the animal contacts the environment (which is unlike most other phenotypic characters). An obvious example of this duality is habitat selection. A number of morphological and behavioural elements contribute to the totality of behaviour that we call habitat selection. All will be a product of evolution. Yet the very act of selecting, that is choosing, a habitat will determine resource availability, predatory pressures and all the other environmental forces that will act upon that animal and which we collectively refer to as selection pressures. This is just another way of saying that selection operates upon the phenotype and since animal phenotypes are active operators upon the world and hence upon selection pressures, the evolutionary paradigm must be expanded to include such active phenotypic intervention. Viewed in this light, the study of behaviour is at the very heart of modern biology and the major achievement of classical ethology and contemporary psychobiology has been to put it there.

Thus we have two vigorous and expanding areas of behavioural study. But what exactly is the relationship between brain-behaviour studies and behavioural biology? More pertinently, what *should* the relationship be? The aim of this chapter is to consider how these key areas relate to one another, and the extent to which at least some degree of combined approach can overcome some of the criticisms and some of the conceptual problems which each faces as a separate discipline. The potential for adding to our understanding of behaviour, the brain and evolutionary biology is enormous, provided that we are circumspect and thoughtful and avoid some of the errors of the past eras of psychobiology (Lockard, 1971).

The two cultures of biology

It is often said that biologists fall into one of two camps or 'cultures'. Mayr (1958) has consistently presented this distinction in terms of the nature of the question posed by the scientist. On the one hand, there are evolutionary biologists who are concerned with the survival value of attributes and of their phylogenetic history as this has been shaped by natural selection. (It should be noted that technically survival value must be translated into reproductive competence or fitness – there are some animals that die during or soon after the act of reproduction!) Such biologists are inclined to ask 'why' in the sense of 'what was or is the functional value of this attribute to this organism'. For example, the relatively great size of the cerebral neocortex in certain orders of mammals (notably carnivores and primates) may be considered in terms of the value of this part of the brain to these kinds of animals (see Chapters 6 and 7 of this volume). On the other hand, there are process biologists whose principal concern is with processes and mechanisms without regard to history or functional value. These biologists ask mainly 'how' questions. To continue with our example of mammalian neocortex, the major part of our knowledge of this part of the brain derives from process approaches such as the anatomical projections to and from circumscribed areas, or the relationships which have been established between the electro-physiological properties of such areas and the behavioural deficits consequent upon their removal.

'How' and 'why' are not the only questions that biologists ask. Tinbergen (1963), for example, has put forward four distinct areas of research in the study of behaviour rather than just two. None the less it is not excessively simple-minded to suggest that most biological work is either of the evolutionary or process kind. There are exceptions. For example, Miller (1977) used complex chromosomal and molecular genetic methods (process biology) to establish the phylogenetic relationships of the great apes and man (evolutionary biology). But even this kind of work, it could be argued, fails as a synthesis of process and evolutionary biology because all that it does is use the tools of one culture to address an issue in the other. Indeed a hardline view is that since each culture asks different questions and thus receives different answers, they will always remain separate; the Miller work, which we will call a combinative study, is the kind that gets as close as one ever will to a marriage of the two. If this is the case, are there any equivalent combinative studies of behaviour which involve manipulation or measurement of brain function and which are cast within an evolutionary context, or evolutionary studies of behaviour which have utilized brain manipulation?

In order to supply a partial answer to this question, a brief survey was carried out on four journals. The journals were chosen because two of them are major outlets for brain-behaviour reports (*Journal of Comparative and Physiological Psychology* and *Physiology and Behaviour*) and the other two are traditional places for the publication of ethologic-evolutionary studies (*Animal Behaviour* and *Zeitschrift für Tierpsychologie*). Only the output of one recent year was examined (1977 in all cases except for the *Zeitschrift* where 1976 was used), and a study was defined as combinative by its use of concepts or methods from one culture to investigate a problem in the other. Consider the following examples. Drinking is a behaviour which is not only non-arbitrary but exceedingly important for survival. However, a study which reports upon the lesion effects of certain brain structures on drinking behaviour is in spirit and intention purely process biology because its concern is the elucidation of the neurological basis of a very widespread behaviour. A paper which reports the effects of hormonal release from a certain part of the brain on the behaviour of urine-marking, on the other hand, is a combinative study. This is because the behaviour used is highly species-specific and known to have a certain functional value to that animal and perhaps a few related species. It can therefore be classed as evolutionary biology whereas the hormonal question is one of process biology. These examples give the flavour of the basis for the judgements made. Let us consider what the survey found, bearing in mind that others using slightly different criteria for combinative study would have arrived at slightly different figures from those given below, but there is no reason to expect that the differences would be significant.

No single study in *Animal Behaviour* or *Zeitschrift für Tierpsychologie* conformed to a combinative study as described above, though these journals did carry several reports which utilized anatomical and physiological systems other than the brain within an evolutionary framework. In *Physiology and Behaviour* only 1 in 228 reports was a combinative study concerned with the effects of amygdala lesions on intraspecific aggression in Iguanid lizards and in the *Journal of Comparative and Physiological Psychology* 14 of 128 reports used behaviours and notions from evolutionary biology in the study of brain mechanisms.

The point which is being made is not one of condemning the journals cited – their editorial policies are well known and scientists submit their papers to journals which have a tradition of publishing similar work. The point is simply the remarkable degree of segregation between brain-behaviour work and those studies of behaviour which are cast within the framework of evolutionary biology.

Although a degree of segregation is to be expected, the extent to which it currently occurs is unhealthy. I will now argue that some evolutionary studies of behaviour give rise to certain conceptual difficulties which could be considerably alleviated by the appropriate use of brain-behaviour methods, and further that for the neurosciences, brain-behaviour studies are the major route by which contact with evolutionary biology can be made. Thus there is a need for more combinative studies than are being carried out at present. However, it is necessary first to consider the nature of evolutionary theory as a science.

The nature of evolutionary theory

There are very few biologists, if any, who do not accept, in general terms, the theory of evolution. This statement applies to process biologists as well as to evolutionary biologists. It is as well to note that there is argument as to the adequacy of evolution as a formal theory (see, for example, Peters, 1976, for recent discussion of this issue) though this is largely a metatheoretical debate and is not of direct concern to us here. What does matter is the kind of evidence which behavioural studies do and should gather within an evolutionary context and how this relates to one's view of the nature of evolutionary theory.

Simple and concise definitions of evolution are hard to come by. But if one accepts evolution as being descent with modification, the modification being based on the effects of natural selection acting on genotypic and phenotypic variance, and if one accepts reproductive success (that is, descent without regard, for our purposes here, as to whether it is achieved by large numbers of offspring, intensive parental care, or whatever) as being the principal or even only measure of fitness, then it can be argued that there are no direct studies either of the evolution of behaviour or of the effects of behaviour on evolution. This is for two reasons. First, whatever the nature of the study, the final step – that is, the demonstration of a direct link between the behaviour in question and reproductive success – is either entirely lacking, or at best very insecure and tentative in terms of the data. The closest that one comes are studies such as those of Tinbergen et al. (1963) which showed a direct relationship to exist between egg-shell removal from the nest by gulls and degree of predation suffered by the nest. The inference that egg-shell removal is thus directly related to reproductive success is a very small one, but it is an inference none the less. The actual demonstration of the relationship was not made (Tinbergen, 1963). Second, because there is no substantive fossil evidence which bears on the evolution of behaviour, historical reconstruction of behaviour is replete with educated guesswork. For these two reasons, the argument runs, we have an expanding area of science which the purist might claim fails because of a lack of congruence between its stated aims and the evidence that it gathers. This argument is wrong, however, because it is based on too narrow a view of the role of evolutionary theory in biological science.

In the sense of the purposes served by evolutionary theory there are, in fact, two forms of theory. In both cases, evolutionary theory is the central concept which makes into a coherent whole widely differing biological disciplines. In the first form of theory, each discipline attempts to establish an explicit hypothetico-deductive and hence predictive base fully capable of matching its aims and its evidence. An example in the area of ecology is Perrin's (1965) work on the relationship between numbers of offspring and availability of food. Another example, this time from sociobiology, is the relationship between the average degree of genetic relatedness and forms of social interaction (Wilson, 1975). There is also the weaker, that is broader, predictive statement of the following kind: 'Predators on animals with aposematic marking must be able to associate visual with taste cues.' Not a very exact statement, but a prediction none the less, which together with more detailed work constitutes theory capable of generating predictions.

The second form in which evolutionary theory is used is not really as theory but as a central explanatory concept which acts to organize what is already known into meaningful and coherent patterns. These patterns of information serve the very important function of helping the scientist to distinguish between significant and insignificant fact, or whether a question is a sensible one to ask in the first place. This is using evolutionary theory as explanation without prediction (Scriven, 1959), or what Popper (1972) calls 'generalized historical explanation'. It is in this sense that behaviour is usually described as having functional, i.e. adaptive, value. The general assumption made is that behaviour, like any other phenotypic feature, has an evolutionary history, a history formed by the action of natural selection on behavioural variants with those variants being selected which increase the fitness of the animal. An example of this approach is the work of Bolles (1970) on avoidance learning which postulates the rate of learning how to avoid aversive events as the dimension which distinguishes the study of biologically trivial learning problems (defined by a very extended acquisition) from those which have functional significance for the animal and hence are quickly learned. It does, after all, make sense that learning to avoid dangerous or aversive events should be rapid, and that if it is not then the behaviour under examination is not, in my opinion, worth studying because it is of little importance to the animal in its normal environment. (This does not, of course, condemn work on all forms of prolonged learning, such as the acquisition of motor skills, which occur normally.)

It is in this second form, as explanation, that evolution has been most used by behavioural scientists. Explanation, by definition, is *post hoc* theorizing and such use of evolutionary theory has been criticized for its lack of vigour at best or sheer invalidity at worst (Klopfer, 1973; Wilson, 1975). Yet recently psychology has been castigated for its failure to appreciate modern evolutionary theory at all (Hodos and Campbell, 1969; Lockard, 1971) and so is 'damned if it does and damned if it doesn't'. But if evolution *is* the central conceptual framework of biology, which I believe it is, and if psychology *has* been singularly guilty of failing to incorporate itself into the modern synthesis of evolutionary biology, which it has, then surely it is better that the increasing numbers of behavioural scientists cognizant of evolutionary thinking should use the theory in its broader, if weaker, sense than not to use it at all?

Evolutionary studies of behaviour

For convenience, the approaches to the study of evolution and behaviour will be considered in this chapter as falling into four distinguishable categories. These are the genetics of behaviour, the study of teleonomy or function, behavioural ecology, and the comparative method based on the concept of homology. Some may argue for the existence of more divisions, and others that the distinctions are arbitrary or at least temporary and will disappear in time. Both alternative views are as likely to be correct as the position adopted here. The point of the distinctions made is simply to provide a framework within which the relative strengths and weaknesses of each approach can be discussed, and consideration given to how each might be improved by a closer working relationship with brain-behaviour studies. In fact, we will see that two of these approaches are quite independent of brain-behaviour studies. But considerable advantage can be gained by behaviour genetics and the comparative method if closer links with brain-behaviour work are established. We begin, therefore, with a brief look at functional and ecological studies of behaviour and then consider the remaining approaches at greater length.

Teleonomic studies of behaviour

Teleonomy is a term which was introduced by Pittendrigh (1958) to refer to the study of the adaptiveness of behaviour. He suggested the word teleonomy to describe valid studies of adaptations based on the knowledge or study of the history of selection pressures, including current animal–environment interactions, and the way in which these have moulded phenotypic traits (i.e. essentially historical reconstruction). This is to be distinguished from 'teleology' which is scientifically invalid because the explanation invokes some form of finalism – that is, either the animal or some other force forms the adaptation because it has knowledge of what future adaptive requirements will be. Teleonomic studies of behaviour, broadly, take three forms: first, theoretical, and often speculative, accounts of the evolutionary origins of behaviour and psychological processes such as non-verbal communication (Bateson, 1968), intelligence (Rozin, 1976) and learning (Plotkin and Odling-Smee, 1979); second, there are descriptive studies of behaviour of free-living animals and the way in which this behaviour appears to be moulded to the requirements of the environment, one of the most classic of such studies being the work of Cullen (1957) on the cliff-nesting behavioural adaptations of the kittiwake; and finally there are studies in which the intervention of the observer (who, in effect, becomes an experimenter) seeks to establish the adaptive nature of behaviour by considering its consequences, as in the Tinbergen et al. (1963) study on egg-shell removal by black-headed gulls.

Hinde (1975) has discussed this approach at length and argues that the principal weakness of such work lies in most studies demonstrating, or arguing, only a weak case (what the behaviour 'does') rather than focussing upon the strong case (the consequences of the behaviour in terms of differential reproduction being contingent upon that behaviour). Brain-behaviour studies have little help to offer here. Indeed, although some scientists have extended their thinking to incorporate a teleonomic approach to brain-behaviour relations, as in Jerison's (1973) writings on the relationship between brain size and intelligence or that of Diamond and Hall (1969) regarding the function of neocortex in 'primitive' mammals such as the hedgehog, such work never involves actual demonstrations of differential reproductive success as a consequence of the functions concerned. Thus they suffer from the same weakness as the purely behavioural studies.

Behavioural ecology

A bleak future has recently been predicted for physiological psychology (Wilson, 1975). Clearly I do not believe this to be the case since the rationale behind this chapter is to sketch the important role that brain-behaviour studies have in evolutionary biology. However, it is significant that the prediction came from the quarter that it did. Ecological studies of behaviour are based on understanding the 'rules of the evolutionary game as it is played in the ecological theatre' (Klopfer, 1973, p. 117) with some theorists insisting on the central place of genetics in such an approach (for example, Wilson, 1975) whilst others (such as Crook et al., 1976) have argued against the need for genetic evidence. An interesting, highly successful and expanding approach in its own right, the ecological study of behaviour has neither conceptual nor historical links with brain-behaviour studies. But, of course, it does not follow from this that the latter is doomed as a science. There is a strong case to be made for some contemporary physiological psychology being condemned as behaviourally, morphologically and biologically trivial, and for a marked lack of theory, as will be suggested towards the end of this chapter. It would be silly, however, to throw the baby out with the bathwater. Especially when the infant, even if not as young as is seemly in one still unable to bath itself, has such an important future role.

Behaviour genetics

The genetics of behaviour is the cornerstone of evolutionary studies of behaviour. Dobzhansky's assertion that 'All bodily structures and functions, without exception, are products of heredity realized in some sequence of environments. So also are all forms of behaviour, also without exception' (Dobzansky, 1972, p. 530) now has a firm empirical foundation (see Chapter 1). There is no reason to doubt the general truth of the assertion, and behaviour genetics will continue to grow as an important area of evolutionary-behavioural research. But this is not to minimize the difficulties which the area faces, difficulties which have been most recently and extensively reviewed by Manning (1975) and to which brain-behaviour studies may have something to contribute in terms of resolving some of these problems.

Manning's review points to five problems confronted by behaviour genetics, especially as these bear directly upon evolutionary issues.

62 Brain, Behaviour and Evolution

Three of these, it will be argued here, cannot be resolved by brain-behaviour studies, but the other two can be assisted by such work.

(1) The selection practised in the laboratory is often, unwittingly, for traits other than those originally intended. Thus in Tryon's early studies on maze-bright and dull rats the results were attributable to selecting for the capacity to learn kinaesthetic information, and our understanding of maze intelligence was not advanced, except insofar as it be, in fact, a susceptibility to kinaesthetic information. Manning points out that selection acts as an opportunistic system which cares little for the means by which the end is attained. Evolutionists have long recognized the difficulties this raises for understanding the precise mechanics of evolution (Pittendrigh, 1958), and this is a particularly acute problem when the traits under investigation are behavioural. For example, one of the most pressing problems faced by any animal is 'knowing' to what species it belongs in order to avoid wasteful gamete exchange and loss. In this instance the end is knowledge regarding who is a member of one's own species, or which products originate with a member of one's own species. In birds, for example, the means by which this can be done range from highly preprogrammed recognition of species characteristics through to early learning (so-called imprinting) and on to very complex and subtle interactions between genetic, experiential and learning factors which result in the appearance of dialect in birdsong of certain species, and the role that dialect plays in the mating behaviour of these birds. Thus own-species recognition, as a pivotal point of the role of behaviour in the evolutionary process, can be achieved in a number of different ways, and lacking direct experimental evidence it is never possible to make assumptions with any certainty as to exactly how it is being achieved.

(2) A related problem is the validity of the behaviours and behavioural measures used in the laboratory. That is, how congruent are the behaviours studied with those which are normally subject to selection pressures under free-living conditions? There is always the possibility that the behaviours studied are gross and/or trivial, again sometimes inadvertently as, e.g., when the effects of selection on nest-building turns out to be due to the thickness of fur rather than an effect on behaviour *per se*. It should be noted that not only is physiological psychology not of any assistance in solving this particular problem, but it is subject to similar criticism, arguably in stronger form. This point will be returned to below when we go on to consider some of the short-comings of brain-behaviour studies.

(3) There is an unknown degree of developmental plasticity in most behaviour traits. This means that ascertaining the way genetic units map into behavioural units is an immensely difficult task. The seemingly high degree of specificity shown by honey bees, where single genes have been shown to control discrete behaviours of uncapping cells in the hive and removing dead or diseased larvae, is rare. It is also probably an illusion of simplicity since it is likely that these single genes control systems which are themselves controlled by many genes (Manning, 1975). The general rule which seems to govern the relationship between genes and behaviour is one:many and many:one mapping of genotypic to phenotypic units.

In these three cases, brain-behaviour studies have little assistance to offer to behavioural genetics. There are, however, two further problems where there is much to be gained by collaborative genetic-physiological and physiologic-behavioural approaches in unravelling the evolution of behaviour.

(4) Both Manning, and earlier Atz (1970), point to the difficulties that we will have until such time as it is possible to establish biologically valid behavioural units. The problem is very simply that behaviour is a continuing stream of animal–environment interactions and it is difficult to know, without being arbitrary and hence unmeaningful, where one behaviour ends and another begins. Thus the problem of behavioural unitization is one of being able to define, and so measure, behaviours which occur in the free-living animal. These behaviours need not necessarily be stereotyped in form though of course they may well be so, and they will derive from a knowledge of 'stop-start' limits or markers. These might take the form of the appearance of a releaser or sign stimulus (for example, an event moving within certain rate and size limits across the visual field of a toad) as the 'start' marker and the consummatory act (swallowing the prey by the toad) as the 'stop' marker to define what classical ethologists would call a fixed or modal action pattern of predation. Alternative forms of markers might be conditional or discriminative stimuli on the one hand and conditional or unconditional responses on the other. There are two important reasons why such unitization must be achieved. First, comparative studies only become possible when one can be certain that what is being compared between different animals *is*, in fact, the 'same' behaviour. We will return to this aspect of the problem later when discussing the concept of homology. Second, the problem is vital to the study of the genetics

of behaviour in that whilst the genetic units can be defined in terms of chromosomes, nucleotide sequences or cistrons, it is necessary to have behavioural units to which the genetics can be related. In empirical terms, statements on the genetic bases of behaviour only have meaning when we know exactly what behaviour is being referred to. So if we have no units of behaviour then we have no way of tracing the development of phenotypic behaviours from genotypic characters. In other words, the way to an effective science of behavioural genetics is blocked by a lack of such behavioural unitization.

There are several possible ways of overcoming this difficulty. As already indicated, one can follow classical ethology and adopt the 'fixed' or 'modal' action pattern whose limits are defined by the occurrence of a releaser on the one hand and the appropriate consummatory response on the other. But the action pattern is a notion which itself has problems. Notably, which releaser does actually control the onset of the act, and which consummatory response is appropriate to which releaser are both uncertain issues and directly concern the problem of unitization itself. Alternatively, if the behaviour is learned and the learning conforms to the conditioning paradigm, then unitization by way of conditional stimulus onset and conditional response termination might work. Unfortunately, instances of pure classical conditioning are notoriously difficult to observe within the context of normal free-living behaviour. Further, if the learning is of the instrumental or operant form then it is frequently impossible to isolate the discriminative stimulus which controls the behavioural sequence.

A third possibility is suggested by Manning (1975). This is to support one's definition of a behavioural unit, whatever it is, with neurological data. Bentley and Hoy have done precisely this using cricket song as the action pattern (Bentley and Hoy, 1974). They found that the song of these insects exactly reflected the firing patterns of motor neurons in specifiable parts of the nervous system, and that distinctive genotypes have neurons which fire in distinctive patterns. In short, they had demonstrated the existence of behaviourally specifiable units which correlate highly with physiologically specifiable units. Unfortunately, every feature of song studied by Bentley and Hoy proved to be polygenically controlled and so specification of the genetic units proved impossible. Another instance of work along these lines is that of Ikeda and Kaplan (1974) who demonstrated the relationship between a pattern of leg-shaking in *Drosophila melano-*

gaster which is specific to a single-mutant gene and the activity of neurons in specific regions of the thoracic ganglion. In this latter case, unfortunately, the behaviour is not clearly related to normal action patterns in this species. However both examples make a simple but powerful point. If the need is for well-demarcated, quantifiable behavioural units, then neurological correlates may be of assistance either in establishing what exactly these units are in the first instance, or in confirming the validity of already known behavioural data.

(5) Last but perhaps the biggest difficulty of all to the behavioural geneticist: 'how is behavioural potential itself represented in genetic terms?' (Manning, 1975, p. 80). This is one of the central problems of behavioural biology and is reminiscent of Schneirla's (1956) warning, as part of the argument as to whether any behaviour can be thought of as being entirely genetic in origin, that genes are a very long way away from behaviour. Manning is acutely aware of this difficulty and offers nervous system structure and function as at least a partial solution. That is, if the distance separating genes from behaviour is both conceptually and empirically very great, then a consideration of the structural substrata of behaviour as a way-station between genes and behaviour as a phenotypic trait is a possible means of breaking the problem down into manageable proportions.

Replacing a larger 'mind-gene' problem with the two lesser difficulties of 'brain-gene' and 'mind-brain' may at first sight appear to be no kind of solution at all. However, our habitual mode of thought by which we seem to group genes and brains together as structures makes the first transition conceptually simple, even if it is in fact anything but easy both in terms of the mechanisms involved and the current paucity of empirical knowledge. Thus, for example, the problem of moving from a genotype to a brain which is deficient in the production of a certain neurotransmitter substance in some particular region (see Chapter 4) does not appear to be great – genes control the production of enzymes, enzymes determine the way in which cells are built and function, and specialized parts of nerve cells are known to be involved in neurotransmitter production. The second transition, that from brain to behaviour is, of course, the very substance of brain-behaviour studies and, appallingly complex empirical difficulties apart, is a well-established scientific discipline.

Furthermore, the use of nervous system structure and function as just such a way-station in gene-behaviour problems has already been pioneered in the studies already mentioned concerning song production and reception in the cricket and leg movements in the fruitfly. So compelling are these studies both in terms of overall conception and elegance of data that they suggest that the case be most strongly stated as follows. Following the demonstration of the genetic basis of some particular behaviour, the next step should be one of establishing the neurological correlates of the genetics (which would restrict such work, at least in its beginnings as is indeed the case, to animals with relatively simple nervous systems). With the morphology as the connecting link, and knowing what behaviour is being dealt with by the initial observation, then using all the techniques available from modern brain-behaviour studies one should proceed to establish the way in which the behaviour is generated by the neural structures in question. In this way, studying the neurological correlates of behaviour becomes an integral part of behaviour genetics.

The homology of behaviour

Phenotypic characters in different species of animals are said to be homologous if they share a common ancestry (for example, the wings of bats and birds, the shared ancestors being stem reptiles) but are analogous if they only have the same function (as, for example, the wings of bats and insects, where the common ancestry of vertebrates and arthropods is too remote to allow for meaningful comparison). The study of homologous characters was central to comparative anatomy of the late-nineteenth century and much of the first half of this century and was the principal tool both by which the evolutionary relationships of animals were worked out, as well as knowledge gained about changes in structures as a response to changing selection pressures. An explicit assumption of classical ethology has been that behaviour, like the study of anatomy, can be subjected to comparative analysis using the tool of homology and that in so doing not only would the evolution of behaviour come to be understood in the same kind of detail as, say, the vertebrate forelimb, but behavioural homologies might be useful in establishing phylogenetic relatedness when other criteria failed.

Classical ethologists seem never seriously to have questioned either the validity of the concept itself, which is not our concern here, or whether the concept could be properly applied to behaviour. Recently serious questions have been raised regarding the applicability of homology to the study of behaviour (Atz, 1970; Klopfer, 1973; Hodos, 1976). Briefly, these are as follows:

(1) Homology only applies to structure, or to functions whose structures are known. Behaviour, however, is habitually treated as abstracted function without regard to structure by most scientists, and even those currently working on attempting to establish the structural substrata of behaviour do not yet know enough to be able to supply a structural account for any significant form of behaviour.

(2) The lack of an adequate unitization of behaviour means that it is never possible to be certain that homologous units are being compared, and therefore that observed differences are due to real evolutionary divergence rather than merely being the result of different characters being mistakenly compared.

(3) For both of the above reasons, and because behaviour leaves no appreciable fossil record, the comparative method in behaviour relies upon the prior establishment of phylogenetic relatedness using other homologous phenotypic characters. Thus subsequent analysis of behavioural homologies is circular.

The impact of brain-behaviour studies, work which by definition seeks to establish the morphological substrata of behaviour, on the study of behavioural homology is immediately obvious. Reconsider each of the above points of criticism in turn:

(1) Though ethologists have, by and large, insisted that behaviour be viewed as structure, they have never been explicit as to why this is possible. The answer lies in the definition of any structure as an entity whose component parts bear a relatively invariant relationship to one another. Thus any relatively stereotyped behaviour, be it a reflex, an orienting response or a fixed action pattern, is indeed a structure and any additional objections to seeing behaviour as structure, such as the impermanence of behaviour and problems of recording and analysis, are technical matters and not serious theoretical objections. (It is the opinion of this writer that a much larger proportion of behaviour is stereotyped, even in man, than is generally assumed. The impression of extreme behavioural flexibility derives both from simply ignoring that very great mass of behaviour ranging from pupillary reflexes and sneezing to walking and sitting which is manifestly stereotyped and structured, and also from our losing sight of the way in which even our most treasured forms of flexibility, i.e. language and reasoning, are themselves structures. The argument becomes more complex than is allowed in this chapter, but the reader

is advised to consider seriously what proportion of his or her behaviour is truly new, or even just a little new, each time it occurs.) If this line of argument is correct and behaviour is as much structure (in time) as skeletal elements are (in space), then the objection to the use of homology is invalid. But if it continues to be felt that in some way behaviour is different from other phenotypic characters and cannot be treated as structure in its own right, then brain-behaviour studies must increasingly reveal the morphological substrata of behaviour and the objection to the use of homology becomes simply that at the moment we just do not know enough. If brain-behaviour studies continue at their present rate of production then it must be the case that it is merely a matter of time before this main criticism disappears.

(2) The formidable problem of the unitization of behaviour has already been discussed regarding behaviour genetics. Brain-behaviour work has, it will be remembered, an important part to play in establishing valid behavioural units.

(3) History cannot be reversed, and if we already know a great deal about the phylogenetic relationships of extant species then we would be foolish not to use that knowledge, even if one then risks accusations of circular reasoning and methods. This issue aside, however, a successful brain-behaviour science must ultimately overcome this third criticism of the use of homology in that recourse then need not necessarily be had to irrelevant morphological features such as skeletal structure to decide which animals should be compared with one another. In theory, neurological structures are available for such use, and knowing what behaviours they subserve all traces of circularity in the making of comparisons disappear.

In summary, brain-behaviour work has much to offer in solving the problems of the study of behavioural homology. We can now begin to consider whether the right kind of studies are being carried out.

Brain-behaviour studies within the context of evolutionary biology

It has already been indicated that few biologists, whatever the nature of their work, doubt the general 'truth' of modern evolutionary theory, even though, as with any living theory, it will continue to change as further knowledge is acquired and new concepts adopted to cope with an expanding area of science. Historically, none the less, psychological and physiological studies of behaviour have been firmly a part of process biology and it remains the case that large numbers of neuroscientists and psychologists continue to think that an evolutionary perspective has little to offer either in terms of creating a powerful empirical framework or in establishing strong theories of behaviour. The remainder of this chapter will examine some examples of work which have been influenced by aspects of evolutionary biology, and then consider the reverse side of the coin to the previous section, i.e. the advantages to brain-behaviour work in particular and to neuroscience in general of a more explicitly evolutionary approach.

Brain-behaviour studies directly influenced by evolutionary biology

The following is by no means an exhaustive survey and is intended merely to give some selected examples of work covering a wide range of topics and methods. It must be reiterated, however, that the total amount of such work being done, as seen in the sampling for combinative studies presented earlier, is a very small proportion of the massive output of brain-behaviour studies reported over the last twenty years.

Genetic-physiological studies These, such as that of Bentley and Hoy, have already been mentioned. Suffice it to say that such work presents a powerful synthesis of methods which should come to play an increasingly central role in biological studies of behaviour.

Experiments guided by the comparative method Despite the strong claim that such studies have for contributing to knowledge of behavioural homology, remarkably few efforts have been directed quite explicitly to the comparative study of brain-behaviour relationships. Let us consider just two of these which illustrate some of the problems inherent in this area. Delacour and Borst (1972) lesioned the 'same' region of the thalamus (the centrum-medianum and parafascicular complex – see Chapter 2) in three species, namely the rat, cat and Irus macaque monkey. They also used the 'same' behavioural tests for all animals, i.e. the effects of such lesions on responsiveness to electric shock, and acquisition and retention of two-way active avoidance learning. They found that the lesion effects, which are reasonably well known in the rat, could not be demonstrated in the other two species. While the results are quite clear, the interpretation of the findings is exceedingly difficult and typifies comparative behavioural studies which use relatively unrelated, if conveniently available, species (drawn in this case from three different orders). First, there is the problem of anatomical definition. The vertebrate brain is several orders of magnitude more complex structurally than is the skeleton, and there is no certainty that the thalamic complex lesioned by Delacour and Borst has the same anatomical boundaries in three relatively unrelated species. Indeed what defines neurological structure is itself a vexed issue, and is most likely a complex of afferent and efferent projections, within-structure cellular characteristics (cytoarchitectonics), neurotransmitter features and gross structural position. Had these workers used more closely related species, drawn at least from the same order, or better still from the same family or genus, the anatomical uncertainties would have been much reduced. In short, any differences observed in this study might be due not to different brain-behaviour relationships in the different animals but simply to their having lesioned different regions of the brain – which then reduces the work to a trivial level. Second, there is that complex of interpretative problems concerning comparability of locomotor, motivational, stimulus salience and learning differences, which without the appropriate control procedures (Bitterman, 1965), makes it impossible to ascribe differences in findings to different causes in different species. For example, one species may freeze rather than return to an area where it has previously been subjected to noxious stimulation, whereas another species might not. Very different results would then be found in a two-way avoidance test of learning and the cause would be one of species-typical responding to aversive stimulation (Bolles, 1970). Or it may be as simple as the shock being physically received in different, and more or less painful, ways by animals with different forms of locomotion, posture and so on. Again the use of less diverse species would have reduced the magnitude of these problems, but not necessarily their essence.

Masterton and Skeen (1972) took a rather different approach. They used three species (the hedgehog, a ground-dwelling insectivore; the tree shrew, an arboreal insectivore; and the bushbaby, a prosimian primate) which could on taxonomic grounds be better justified as they form an approximation to early mammalian lineage. Using anatomical techniques they compared the size of the prefrontal system of the nucleus medialis dorsalis of the thalamus, its cortical projection in prefrontal cortex, and the caudate nucleus which is one of the principal efferent projections from prefrontal cortex. All three regions are known to be involved in the performance of tasks with a delay component where, following an exposure to certain stimulus conditions, an interval of time is interposed before the animals are allowed to act on the information which has been received. Lesions of the prefrontal system in primates are known to reduce the delays over which the correct performance can be maintained. Masterton and Skeen did not lesion their animals. They simply correlated performance in the delayed alternation task with the size of the prefrontal system and found a significant correlation to exist. Because they used more closely related species both methodological and interpretative problems relating to anatomical and behavioural differences were greatly reduced. It is possible to conclude, at least tentatively, that the behavioural control of homologous structures of the brain in the test situation studied was the same for all three species.

It is clear from these two studies that comparative brain-behaviour work poses some very considerable difficulties, and that perhaps is why there is such a paucity of these studies in the literature. They combine all of the problems of comparative and physiological experiments in a single package. None the less, their potential, both for providing an underpinning for the study of behavioural homology as well as supplying greatly needed evidence for changing brain-behaviour relations across species, is such that one can only hope that such work will be increasingly undertaken in the future. The classic comparative studies of ethology like that of Lorenz (1972) on dabbling ducks and Tinbergen (1959) on gulls were so rich in detailing differences between species of the same genus, behavioural differences which *must* be expressions of underlying neurological differences, that similar work which adds an explicit brain dimension cannot fail to be of interest and importance. Such studies will be very expensive in terms of time and effort. But then the usefulness of current brain-behaviour comparisons which are largely *post hoc* and arbitrary (for example, experimentation and discussion of the effects of lesions of frontal cortex in those old favourites, the rat, cat and monkey, and their implications for frontal cortex function in man) is so questionable that it seems unlikely that this kind of work, which has consumed vast resources of time and effort from neuroscientists over the last thirty to forty years, will have much place when the history of the unfolding of knowledge of brain-behaviour relationships comes to be written.

Motivation, consummatory behaviour and electrical stimulation of the brain   A significant aspect of behaviour concerns the way it is driven and directed. Traditionally a part of the study of motivation for the psychologist, its ethological equivalent has been the study of consummatory behaviour and elicitation of such drive-reducing activity by particular environmental events termed releasers. This is the area of brain-behaviour relationships which has most directly attracted the attention of ethologists and is one of the few problems which ethology has actively studied by using direct intervention in brain activity. Von Holst and Von Saint-Paul (1963), for example, showed that electrical stimulation of certain areas of the brain of domestic chickens elicited fixed action patterns and consummatory acts which were both a part of the natural behavioural repertoire of these birds and also tended to be appropriate to the stimulus conditions of the environment at the time of stimulation. Thus electrical stimulation of a fixed level and in some specific brain region would elicit restless locomotion in the absence of any external threat stimulus, but if a model of some usual predator was presented during such stimulation then immediate attack behaviour would be elicited, which would not have occurred prior to brain stimulation.

The elicitation of consummatory behaviour by brain stimulation is a well-established phenomenon (see Carlson, 1977, ch. 16, for a recent review). Work with a common conceptual basis is that on the effects of hormone levels on nest-building and egg-brooding behaviour in birds, or the retrieval behaviour of lactating rodent mothers. In all cases one is concerned with the neurological bases of species-specific behaviours, especially as these manifest themselves in consummatory acts. Glickman and Schiff (1967) have taken the boldest step along this particular road by suggesting that what psychologists refer to as a reinforcement and what ethologists term consummatory behaviour are identical and subserved by activity in specific brain-stem circuits.

Brain-behaviour studies using ethologically 'valid' behaviour   One of the outstanding and most unfortunate features of work on brain-behaviour relationships is its predominant use of (a) species which are easily available and convenient rather than their being chosen for their taxonomic status or ecological interest, and (b) behavioural observations and tests which are drawn from the arbitrary conventions of laboratory behavioural studies rather than because they may be related to behaviour which is important under normal free-living conditions. This arbitrary and unreal aspect of physiological psychology is rooted in the history and conventions of a science whose origins are entirely within the traditions of process biology. It has recently, however, become increasingly apparent that results either change, become more or less pronounced or, most importantly, their interpretation assumes a quite different complexion when placed within the perspective of evolutionary biology.

Contrast the pessimism of Gaito (1976) who concludes that the biochemical studies of the macromolecular bases of memory have been largely a waste of time and the steady flow of results from Bateson (1976) and his colleagues. Gaito is quite correct. But why should so many scientists working with great enthusiasm and the vision of another breakthrough along the lines of the cracking of the genetic code have come up with so little? The answer, I think, is that unlike genetics which had almost a century of research and accumulating knowledge behind it as to where to look and what to look for, the biochemical work on memory was premature. Nobody yet knows where to look for the effects of learning of the sort generally used in these studies, i.e. the arbitrary conditioning and instrumental learning studies of conventional psychology which have been absorbed into the brain-behaviour laboratories. Nor does anyone know what information is being stored since there is absolutely no evidence upon which to base the assumption that what animals do learn about is simply mapped out from a knowledge of the laboratory paradigms. In short, most of the work on the biochemical bases of memory had been done in the absence of knowledge as to where to look and what to look for. Bateson's studies have had a much firmer base. They used imprinting as the form of learning, and imprinting is a 'valid' rather than arbitrary situation to use because it is known to occur in certain species of birds and at a certain point in their development. Further, by restricting themselves to the visual modality they were able to narrow down the areas where macromolecular effects might be detected. Exactly how far the Bateson studies will take knowledge in this area is a matter for the future, and whether their possible success will be due to the use of imprinting is debatable, but the difference between the decline of such work in almost all quarters except that of the chick imprinting project is marked.

Contrast again the unexpected learning capacity which has been demonstrated by Oakley (see Chapter 7) with the totally decorticate rabbit and rat. Yet these same animals with massive cerebral lesions cannot or do not perform what most neuroscientists would judge to be a much simpler act, i.e. copulation. The cause of this deficiency has yet to be ascertained, but one possibility is that copulation in mammals is elicited and guided by a complex of chemical, visual, tactile, auditory and 'social' stimuli which need to be coordinated and integrated into proper temporal sequences. In short, it suggests that copulation is anything but simple and draws from a complex social behavioural repertoire, and that it is the latter which has provided at least some of the selection pressures behind the expansion of neocortex in mammals (Humphrey, 1976).

What an evolutionary perspective can do for brain-behaviour studies

Implicit in what has already been said is the simple message that there are many serious faults in brain-behaviour studies: their in- heritance from an outmoded comparative psychology of the quite incorrect notion of the phylogenetic scale (Hodos and Campbell, 1969); their use of arbitrary test procedures and cavalier extrapolation from rats or cats to monkeys or men. This extrapolation is a natural consequence of the deep man-orientation of the subject and its loss of touch with evolutionary biology. This in turn has resulted in the conceptual elimination of the possibility of real and irreconcilable differences between different species of animals by constant and blind- ing references to a mythical beast called 'the organism'. All of these faults can and should be eliminated by a large infusion of evolutionary biology.

There is an additional and even more fundamental gain which would accrue to the neurosciences and to biology at large if the level of brain-behaviour studies were raised by its taking greater note of evolutionary biology. Behaviour, as argued in the introduction, is at the centre of evolutionary biology because of its dual role as determiner and consequence of selection pressures acting on the phenotype. Behaviour is also the neurosciences' major route into evolutionary biology, and the neurosciences have become one of the most vigorous and important areas of process biology. Thus the study of brain- behaviour relationships is not only the interface between neuroscience on the one hand and evolutionary studies of behaviour on the other, but it is also because of the pivotal role of behaviour, one of the few areas of biology where a true meeting and synthesis of biology's two cultures can occur. This is a unique and onerous position, certainly not one to be taken lightly and probably not appreciated by most investigators into brain-behaviour relationships.

Conclusion

This chapter has attempted to show how both the evolutionary study of behaviour and brain-behaviour work can mutually profit from a greater degree of awareness of the concepts and problems that each has and increased 'inter-cultural' study. It also presents a recurrent theme, namely that the potential contribution of brain-behaviour studies to biology at large is very great indeed, but will probably only be realized when it ceases to operate around the arbitrary and restricted models and concepts of traditional, man-oriented psychology and physiology.

Note

1 My thanks to Professor A. Manning of Edinburgh University for helpful comment on this chapter.

References

Atz, J. W. (1970) The application of the idea of homology to behaviour. In L. R. Aronson, E. Tobach, D. S. Lehrman and J. S. Rosenblatt (eds) *The Development and Evolution of Behaviour*. San Francisco: Freeman, 53–74.

Bateson, G. (1968) Redundancy and coding. In T. A. Sebeok (ed.) *Animal Communication*. Bloomington: Indiana University Press, 641–56.

Bateson, P. P. G. (1976) Neural consequences of early experience in birds. In P. Spencer Davies (ed.) *Perspectives in Experimental Biology*, Vol. 1. London: Pergamon Press, 411–15.

Bentley, D. and Hoy, R. R. (1974) The neurobiology of cricket song. *Scientific American 231*: 34–44.

Bitterman, M. E. (1965) Phyletic differences in learning. *American Psychologist 20*: 396–410.

Bolles, R. C. (1970) Species-specific defence reactions and avoidance learning. *Psychological Review 77*: 32–48.

Carlson, N. R. (1977) *Physiology of Behaviour*. Boston: Allyn and Bacon.

Crook, J. H., Ellis, J. E. and Goss-Custard, J. D. (1976) Mammalian social systems. *Animal Behaviour 24*: 261–74.

Cullen, E. (1967) Adaptations in the kittiwake to cliff-nesting. *Ibis 99*: 275–302.

Delacour, J. and Borst, A. (1972) Failure to find homology in rat, cat and monkey for functions of a subcortical structure. *Journal of Comparative and Physiological Psychology 80*: 458–68.

Diamond, I. T. and Hall, W. C. (1969) Evolution of neocortex. *Science 164*: 251–62.

Dobzhansky, T. (1972) Genetics and the diversity of behaviour. *American Psychologist 27*: 523–30.

Gaito, J. (1976) Molecular psychobiology of memory: its appearance, contributions and decline. *Physiological Psychology 4*: 476–84.

Glickman, S. E. and Schiff, B. B. (1967) A biological theory of reinforcement. *Psychological Review 74*: 81–109.

Hinde, R. A. (1975) The concept of function. In G. Baerends, C. Beer and A. Manning (eds) *Function and Evolution in Behaviour*. Oxford: Clarendon Press, 3–15.

Hodos, W. (1976) The concept of homology and the evolution of behaviour. In R. B. Masterton, W. Hodos and H. Jerison (eds) *Evolution, Brain and Behaviour: Persistent Problems*. Hillsdale: Lawrence Erlbaum, 153–67.

Hodos, W. and Campbell, C. B. G. (1969) Scala naturae. *Psychological Review 76*: 337–50.

Humphrey, N. K. (1976) The social function of intellect. In P. P. G. Bateson and R. A. Hinde (eds) *Growing Points in Ethology*. Cambridge: Cambridge University Press, 303–17.

Ikeda, K. and Kaplan, W. D. (1974) Neurophysiological genetics in Drosophila melanogaster. *American Zoologist 14*: 1055–65.

Jerison, H. J. (1973) *Evolution of the Brain and Intelligence*. London: Academic Press.

Klopfer, P. H. (1973) Does behaviour evolve? *Annals of the New York Academy of Sciences 223*: 113–19.

Lockard, R. B. (1971) Reflections on the fall of comparative psychology. *American Psychologist 26*: 168–79.

Lorenz, K. (1972) Comparative studies on the behaviour of Anatinae. In P. H. Klopfer and U. P. Hailman (eds) *Function and Evolution of Behaviour*. Reading, Mass: Addison-Wesley, 231–59.

Manning, A. (1975) Behaviour genetics and the study of behavioural evolution. In G. Baerends et al. (eds) *Function and Evolution in Behaviour*. Oxford: Clarendon Press, 71–91.

Mason, W. A. and Lott, D. F. (1976) Ethology and comparative psychology. *Annual Review of Psychology*: 129–54.

Masterton, B. and Skeen, L. C. (1972) Origins of anthropoid intelligence. *Journal of Comparative and Physiological Psychology 81*: 423–33.

Mayr, E. (1958) Behaviour and systematics. In A. Roe and G. G. Simpson (eds) *Behaviour and Evolution*. New Haven: Yale University Press, 341–62.

Miller, D. A. (1977) Evolution of primate chromosomes. *Science 198*: 1116–24.

Perrin, C. M. (1965) Population fluctuations and clutch size in the great tit. *Journal of Animal Ecology 34*: 601–47.

Peters, R. H. (1976) Tautology in evolution and ecology. *The American Naturalist 110*: 1–12.

Pittendrigh, C. (1958) Adaptation, natural selection and behaviour. In A. Roe and C. G. Simpson (eds) *Behaviour and Evolution*. New Haven: Yale University Press, 390–416.

Plotkin, H. C. and Odling-Smee, F. J. (1979) Learning, change and evolution. In press in *Advances in the Study of Behaviour 10*.

Popper, K. R. (1972) *Objective Knowledge*. Oxford: Clarendon Press.

Rozin, P. (1976) The evolution of intelligence and access to the cognitive unconscious. *Progress in Psychobiology and Physiological Psychology 6*: 245–80.

Schneirla, T. C. (1956) Interrelationship of the innate and the acquired in instinctive behaviour. In P. P. Grasse (ed.) *L'Instinct dans le comportement des animaux et de l'homme*. Paris: Masson, 387–452.

Scriven, M. (1959) Explanation and prediction in evolution theory. *Science 130*: 477–82.

Seligman, M. E. P. and Hager, J. L. (1972) *Biological Boundaries of Learning*. New York: Appleton-Century-Crofts.

Tinbergen, N. (1959) Comparative studies of the behaviour of gulls. *Behaviour 15*: 1–70.

Tinbergen, N. (1963) On aims and methods of ethology. *Zeitschrift für Tierpsychologie 20*: 410–33.

Tinbergen, N., Broekhuisen, G. J., Feekes, F., Houghton, J. C. W., Kruuk, H. and Szulc, E. (1963) Egg shell removal by the black-headed gull. *Behaviour 19*: 74–117.

Von Holst, E. and Von Saint-Paul, U. (1967) On the functional organization of drives. *Animal Behaviour 11*: 1–20.

Wilson, E. O. (1975) *Sociobiology*. Cambridge Mass.: The Belknap Press.

4 Chemical systems of the brain and evolution

Gaylord D. Ellison

While the principles of evolution have implications for a variety of scientific disciplines, they have had a special impact on the neurosciences. This is because a central theme of evolution is the increasingly more sophisticated methods of adaptability produced by successive generations. Consequently considerations based on evolutionary principles are a fruitful source of speculation about the functional organization of the brain. The central nervous system, with the brain as its head ganglion, has developed as the great controller and co-ordinator of the various physiological functions of the body and of the behavioural patterns by which animals meet the many needs which must be satisfied for survival.

But evolutionary biology can also learn much from the neurosciences. While the vertebrate brain has undergone a series of stages of evolutionary development, its most primitive parts have changed the least during evolution. Yet these same primitive brainstem regions have been the subject of considerable recent investigation using powerful scientific tools such as those developed by modern neurochemistry. It seems likely that from the detailed analysis of the primitive brain of modern animals, information about earlier forms will emerge, for just as bone structure can provide clues as to the ecological niche inhabited by an animal, so too can brain structure and function. Biochemical differences in the brain represent a major way of classifying and distinguishing functional subsystems. In the following section some principles of neurotransmission and of research tools in neuro-chemistry will be reviewed, followed by some implications of recent advances using these techniques.

Chemical neurotransmission

The principal building block of the nervous system is the specialized cell known as the neuron. Neurons have developed to an extreme the ability to depolarize briefly in response to various conditions, and use these brief depolarizations (called 'impulses' or 'spikes' when recorded electrically) as a principal means for encoding information. From a central cell body each neuron sends out processes which connect, or synapse, with other neurons. It is through synapses that messages are passed from nerve cell to nerve cell and information is transformed, eventually to be relayed to the motor system for action.

Chemical transmission at synapses is one of the most consistent characteristics of the vertebrate nervous system, although purely electrical synapses have been found in certain specialized cases such as the electrical organ of eels or certain invertebrate synapses. Chemical transmission involves the release of a small amount of a chemical substance, called the neurotransmitter, from a cell when that cell depolarizes. This neurotransmitter then diffuses through the local environment until it reaches a second cell, where it acts to induce some alteration in the membrane of the receiving cell. It thereby causes some change in the receiving cell's firing rate, or depolarization threshold, or chemical make-up.

It is important to understand the general mechanisms by which such short-range chemical transmission of information is accomplished, for many types of drug therapies and research methodologies are based on highly specific ways in which chemical transmission can be altered. Figure 4.1 shows a generalized and highly schematic synapse. From a distant cell body (not shown), an axon would project some distance and finally terminate in the presynaptic swelling pictured. Within this presynaptic ending are many synaptic vesicles, usually varying in size from 200–900 Å. These vesicles represent storage packets containing neurotransmitter molecules. When the distant cell fires (i.e. transiently reverses its membrane potential), a brief depolarization travels down the axon and, upon reaching the

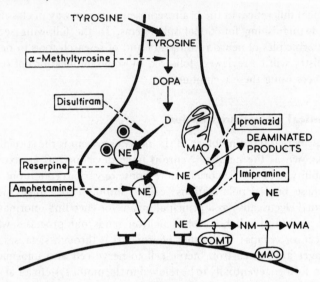

Fig. 4.1   Schematic diagram of a norepinephrine synapse. Tyrosine is taken up by the ending and synthesized to DOPA. This reaction can be blocked by the drug alpha-methyltyrosine. Dopa is further converted to dopamine (D), which is then further converted to norepinephrine (NE) and stored in vesicles. Amphetamine causes the release of stored norepinephrine; some other drugs which alter storage, release or metabolism of NE are shown. MAO = monoamine oxidase; NM = normetanephrine; VMA = 3-methoxy-4-hydroxymendelic acid; and COMT = catechol-O-methyl transferase. Also pictured are a typical reuptake blocker (imipramine), a monoamine oxidase inhibitor, iproniazid, and reserpine which blocks storage. From R. H. Rech and K. E. Moore, *An Introduction to Psychopharmacology.* Copyright 1971 by Raven Press, New York.

presynaptic swelling, causes the release of packets of neurotransmitter. These diffuse across the synaptic cleft (100–500 Å) until they reach the post-synaptic neuron and react with a receptor site situated upon the membrane of the receiving cell. This then induces a change in the membrane potential of the receiving cell and synaptic transmission has occurred. The neurotransmitter molecules can be deactivated or removed from the post-synaptic cell membrane by several means. Local enzymes contained in the region of the synaptic cleft can de-activate the neurotransmitter molecules, thereby terminating the synaptic transmission. Another way of producing this deactivation is for the presynaptic membrane to reabsorb the neurotransmitter back into the presynaptic cell ending, where it can be replaced into synaptic vesicles for future re-use. This method of recycling the neuro-transmitter is called the reuptake process and is very important for some types of neurotransmitters but virtually non-existent in others.

Research tools in neurochemistry

There are a huge number of chemicals present in the brain, but only some of them appear to serve as actual neurotransmitters – others are constituents of membranes or other structural elements, or are contained in non-neural cells such as glia, or act as enzymes related to energy metabolism, nutritional synthesis or neurotransmitter synthesis, and so on. What are the steps by which one can recognize an actual neurotransmitter? The following section will describe

Table 4.1   Possible central nervous system neurotransmitters. Those that are not marked (?) are relatively well established

Monoamines		Peptides	Amino Acids	Others
Indoleamines	*Catecholamines*			
Serotonin	Norepinephrine	Endorphines	γ-aminobutyric	Acetylcholine
Tryptamine (?)	Dopamine	Substance P	acid	Histamine (?)
	Epinephrine (?)	(?)	Glutamic acid (?)	
			Glycine (?)	
			Taurine (?)	
			Aspartic acid (?)	

examples of some of the methodology available in neurochemistry and neuropharmacology. These techniques were actually used to identify four chemicals for which considerable evidence exists indicating usage as central neurotransmitters: acetylcholine (ACh), the ideolamine 5-hydroxytryptamine (5HT, also called serotonin), and two catecholamines: norepinephrine (NE, also known as nora-drenaline) and dopamine (DA). These and several other potential neurotransmitters are listed in Table 4.1. Recent general accounts of neurotransmitters are given in Iversen, Iversen and Snyder (1975), and Iversen and Iversen (1975).

Assays of brain levels

The first step in the discovery of a new brain chemical is usually the development of a method for detecting, reliably identifying and quantifying the presence of the chemical in the brain. This may be a crude spectrophotometric assay, or a highly refined one, such as involving gas–liquid chromatography. Then the regional distribution of the chemical is usually determined by analysing the amount present in various brain regions. Some well-established neurotransmitters, such as ACh, have a widespread distribution throughout the brain, while others, such as DA, are more localized in only a few brain regions. Assays sometimes provide clues as to where the cell bodies of the neurons which use a given neurotransmitter are located. For example, early in the investigation of 5HT it was discovered that when lesions were made in the medial forebrain bundle of rats, the 5HT levels in the higher forebrain dropped to very low levels. This was interpreted as evidence that the cell bodies for 5HT neurons were located somewhere caudal to the lesion, in the brainstem, from which they sent ascending axons which carried 5HT or 5HT-synthesizing enzymes anteriorly, passing through the medial forebrain bundle. This interpretation is now known to be correct.

Microscopic methods

These are methods by which an established neurotransmitter can be selectively stained and then viewed in a light microscope. This is often an extremely powerful step in establishing that a chemical is in fact a neurotransmitter, for a neurotransmitter should be found to be present within cells and is usually concentrated at the ending of axons, in the presynaptic region. In some cases there are no known methods for staining a chemical, as, for example, with ACh. But acetylcholinesterase, the principal enzyme involved in the deactivation of ACh, can be stained and viewed in a microscope. Although this method for localizing ACh neurons is highly indirect and might lead to erroneous conclusions (for example, this same enzyme might also perform other, unrelated functions), it is the best stain available for ACh.

Such a problem is not present in the case of the monoamines NE, DA and 5HT, where an extremely powerful tool has been developed: fluorescence microscopy. This involves obtaining fresh or freeze-dried brain tissue (so that no degradation of brain chemicals has occurred) and reacting it with vapours such as formalin or glyoxylic acid for about an hour at 100° C. Under these conditions the chemical structure of each of these monoamines is modified slightly so as to form a fluorophore (a chemical molecule which, when illuminated by a fluorescent light of a certain wavelength, will reflect back a fluorescence of a different wavelength). Each of these monoamines can be observed directly in a fluorescence microscope when the appropriate histological procedures and filters are used. Because the monoamine is localized within monoamine-containing neurons, what is actually viewed is the cell with all its processes. An interesting variation of these techniques involves the use of antibody staining. Thus, dopamine-beta-hydroxylase (DBH) is the final enzyme involved in the synthesis of NE. One can obtain purified DBH from the adrenal gland of a sheep, inject it into a rabbit, and then obtain antiserum to the foreign DBH from the rabbit blood. This antiserum can be 'tagged' with a fluorescent dye and reacted with fresh brain material. The antibodies will selectively adhere to DBH in the fresh brain, and the location of the DBH can be viewed with a fluorescence microscope. From techniques such as these a high degree of resolution of central neurochemical transmitter systems can be achieved.

Another method for selectively viewing neurochemical systems involves the use of *autoradiography*. At low concentrations, NE molecules are selectively taken up by NE cells (especially by the terminals). This fact can be used to map NE cells and their processes. If one takes a fresh brain section and incubates it for several minutes in an oxygenated buffer solution containing radioactively labelled NE, the labelled NE will selectively accumulate in NE cells, axons and terminals. The brain slice is then dried, perhaps in a freeze dryer to prevent diffusion of the labelled NE out of the cell processes), and then the brain slice is placed against a piece of X-ray film for several weeks in total darkness. When subsequently developed, the X-ray film will be clouded only where labelled NE has accumulated, and the film will therefore picture the distribution of NE uptake and, presumably, NE cells. A powerful variation of this autoradiographic technique involves the injection into the collection of cell bodies in a living animal's brain small amounts of radioactively labelled amino acids. These amino acids will be taken up by cell bodies (but not axons) around the injection site and incorporated into protein molecules as the cell synthesizes material essential for maintenance. At some later time the animal is sacrificed, brain sections are made, placed against X-ray film, and left for several weeks. In this case the clouding of the film will indicate the brain areas to which the cell bodies located in the region of the injection project, for the radio-activity will be transported along axons to terminal regions.

But while the various techniques mentioned above are powerful methods for the study of the anatomical structure of neurotransmitter systems, they are not so useful for determining the *functions* of various neurotransmitter systems – unless the neurotransmitter studied happens to be contained exclusively within an anatomical system with a clear relationship to a certain physiological function, such as the visual system. Furthermore, the relationship of the levels of a given neurotransmitter within the brain to the amount of post-synaptic stimulation produced by that neurotransmitter is often quite complex. For example, if for some reason (such as the presence of a drug or pharmacological agent) the release of a neurotransmitter from pre-synaptic neurons is inhibited or decreased, the amount of that neuro-transmitter present in the brain will often increase gradually (since little of the neurotransmitter is being deactivated). This leads to the paradoxical result of heightened levels but decreased turnover or rate of release. In such cases other research tools are necessary.

Receptor blockers and stimulators

These are pharmacological agents which are usually structurally similar in some aspect of their molecular configuration to an actual neurotransmitter, and which will therefore attach themselves to the receptor sites on the post-synaptic neuron, often more easily than does the neurotransmitter itself. But such a pharmacological agent can have a molecular structure such that it attaches itself to that receptor but does not actually stimulate the receptor. In such a case the net effect will be a blocking of the ability of the actual neurotransmitter to stimulate the post-synaptic neuron. Many such receptor blockers have been discovered for different transmitters. They are often discovered by some biological assay. For example, a frog's heart will continue beating for some time after removal from the frog as long as it is properly oxygenated. The rate of contraction and contractile force of the isolated frog heart will increase appreciably if NE is dripped onto it (this is a sympathetic nervous system response). From the almost random screening of various drugs it was discovered that certain pharmacological agents would, if applied to the frog's heart prior to the application of NE, block the stimulator action of NE. The further refinement of these NE receptor blockers led to the development of several drugs used to treat hypertension in humans.

Conversely, other agents attach themselves to the receptors and actively stimulate them. Such receptor stimulators are often more useful for the study of the actions of neurotransmitters than are the actual neurotransmitters themselves, since they are often much more slowly deactivated by local enzymes and thereby have a considerably prolonged action, and they are often more selective in their actions. Many fruitful studies of brain function have involved the local application of neurotransmitters, receptor blockers and receptor stimulators to discrete regions of the brain through small cannulae implanted directly into crucial brain structures. In other cases it has been possible to measure quantitatively brain receptors by incubating brain preparations with radioactively labelled receptor blockers, washing, and then counting the amount of activity which has been selectively bound to receptors.

Synthesis inhibitors and precursors

Neurotransmitters are synthesized in the brain by a series of enzymatic steps. This can be illustrated by the amino acid tyrosine. Tyrosine is a constituent of many foods. It can cross the blood-brain barrier and, once inside the brain, is taken up by catecholamine-containing neurons. The first step in the ensuing reactions is the conversion of tyrosine to dihydroxyphenylalanine (DOPA) by the enzyme tyrosine hydroxylase. This step is rate-limiting in the synthesis of catecholamines. Next, DOPA is decarboxylated by the enzyme aromatic L-amino acid decarboxylase to dopamine, DA. In DA-containing neurons, the reaction stops here, but in neurons which use NE as their neurotransmitter the DA is further converted by dopamine-β-hydroxylase to NE. Each of these steps in synthesis involves an enzyme, and in some cases it is possible to either deactivate or inhibit the activity of an enzyme by introducing some foreign pharmacological agent. In such a case the levels of the neurotransmitter gradually decrease over time as neurotransmitter is utilized and the synthesis of new transmitter is prevented. The gradual alterations in physiological functions which result are presumably due to preventing normal functions of the neurotransmitter. In other cases it is possible to measure the rate at which neurotransmitter is being utilized. One way of doing this is to inject into the animal a radioactively labelled precursor (such as C^{14} tyrosine) and measure the rate of formation of C^{14} NE. This gives a measure of the rate of the entire reaction, and the effects of stress, for example, on rate of NE synthesis can be studied.

An opposite strategy is to increase transmitter levels by injecting large quantities of a precursor of that neurochemical. For example, DOPA can be injected into an animal. It will cross the blood-brain barrier and then be converted into DA and NE. Resulting alterations in function can then be correlated with the increased catecholaminergic stimulation.

Brain lesions and neurotoxins

A classical way of studying the effects of a neurotransmitter is to determine what alterations are produced when the actions of that neurotransmitter are eliminated. If one knows precisely the location of cell bodies necessary for synthesizing that neurotransmitter, and if they are localized in a brain area, it is possible to produce a discrete lesion (using electrodes and electrical currents) which is confined only to those crucial cell bodies. This would result in the depletion of that transmitter in those areas of the brain to which that region projects. But this method is limited to conclusions only about that particular region of damage, because many neurotransmitters are synthesized

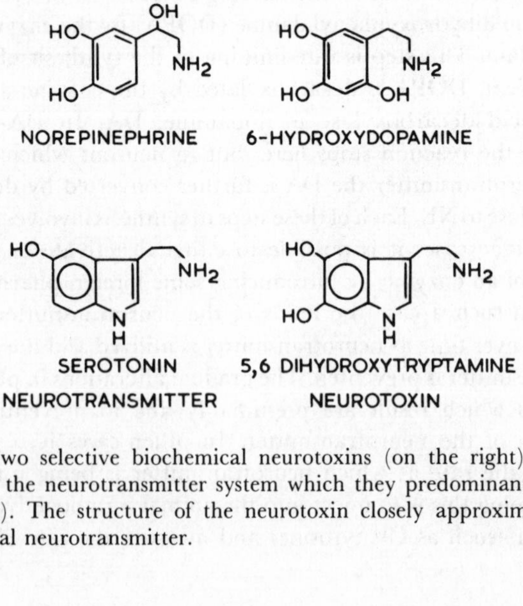

NOREPINEPHRINE   6-HYDROXYDOPAMINE

SEROTONIN   5,6 DIHYDROXYTRYPTAMINE
NEUROTRANSMITTER   NEUROTOXIN

Fig. 4.2   Two selective biochemical neurotoxins (on the right) and the structure of the neurotransmitter system which they predominantly attack (on the left). The structure of the neurotoxin closely approximates that of the normal neurotransmitter.

by cells in several discrete brain regions, which if lesioned would lead to different patterns of depletion of that transmitter. Other transmitters are produced by cells which are exceedingly diffuse in their location in the brain. To deplete such a transmitter, large and widespread lesions must be made, making interpretations difficult because of involvement of other types of lesioned cells.

A more recent development is the discovery of selective neurochemical toxins. These are chemicals which are structurally similar to established neurotransmitters (Figure 4.2), but which are unstable at brain pH and temperature, when they spontaneously auto-oxidize and form toxic compounds such as hydrogen peroxide. When injected into the brain of animals, these compounds are selectively taken up by one neurotransmitter system via the reuptake process since the neurons cannot distinguish between their normal transmitter and the toxin. Widespread biochemical lesions confined to a single neurotransmitter system are produced.

Evolutionary studies of neurotransmitters

The study of how biochemical systems have evolved in the vertebrates is an extremely complex area, for there are almost an infinite combination of techniques available, neurochemical systems and species or brain regions to be studied. Furthermore, the mere detection of a similar neurotransmitter in several divergent species does not necessarily mean that the chemical substance performs any similar functions in the different species or even has any similar evolutionary basis. Neurotransmitters are merely chemical substances which are readily synthesized from available food sources and which have come to be used by the nervous system as messengers. Because many of the common foods on earth contain a few basic amino acids, it seems likely that very different species might evolve the same neurotransmitters through parallel evolution. Thus, it is important to establish not only that a common neurochemical system is present in several different species but that it is produced by homologous anatomical cells, or that it subserves a similar function. This is often difficult or impossible when extremely simple organisms are studied. For example, when protozoan cultures are incubated with radioactively labelled tyrosine for four days, some protozoa, such as the flagellated protozoa *Crithidia fasciculata* and the ciliated protozoa *Tetrahymena pyriformis* have been found to have the capability of converting the tyrosine into the catecholamine NE. It also seems likely that catecholamines subserve some function in these simple organisms, for when Tetrahymena cultures are exposed to reserpine (a drug which causes depletion of the catecholamines) they show decreased growth which is well correlated with the degree of catecholamine depletion (Blum et al., 1966). Other studies have indicated that the monoamines 5HT, NE and DA are present in many flatworms (*Platyhelminthes*) and that these chemicals are not only localized in the cerebral ganglia and ventral nerve cord, but that when histofluorescent techniques are used it can be observed that monoamine-containing cells are generally distributed throughout the organisms' nervous system (Welsh and King, 1970). Yet is is highly unlikely that the common presence of these same chemicals in both extremely simple organisms and in the complex vertebrate brain has any real functional significance.

There are, however, some more complex biochemical methods which do provide correlations between evolutionary development and pharmacology. Consider the tranquillizer benzodiazepam. It is one of the most frequently prescribed tranquillizers in Western Europe and America at the present time: this is because it has a calming action without concurrently depressing higher cortical functions such as thinking, speech and information processing. Where this complex pharmacological agent acts in the brain can be studied using sophisticated receptor binding methods. Brain homogenates are incubated with radioactively labelled diazepam, then washed, and then the radioactivity is counted. Only the radioactivity which is specifically bound to some brain substratum is measured using this technique. When this was done using brain tissue from post-mortem human brains, it was found that the greatest diazepam binding is found in the cerebral cortex, considerably less binding was present in the more primitive limbic forebrain, even less was present in the diencephalon, and binding was extremely low in the hindbrain, including the pons and medulla (see Chapter 2). Thus, there was a good correlation between the degree of tranquillizer binding and recency of evolutionary development within the human brain. This correlation also holds true across a wide variety of species (Nielsen et al., 1978). When the entire head ganglia of invertebrates or the anterior parts of vertebrate brains were dissected and incubated with labelled diazepam, it was found that binding is virtually non-existent in invertebrates such as *Annelida*, *Mollusca*, *Arthropoda* and *Insecta*. In more primitive vertebrates, such as the bony hagfish, binding is also extremely low but it then progressively increases through less primitive fishes, *Amphibia*, *Reptilia*, *Aves*, and finally reaches its greatest levels in *Mammalia*. Thus, it seems likely that as more sophisticated pharmacological agents are developed for human therapeutic uses, the more sophisticated study of evolutionary aspects of biochemical systems will also be possible.

Functional classes of neurotransmitters

Before comparing the effects of neurotransmitters in different species, it is necessary to consider what types of neurochemical transmitters lend themselves to this type of analysis. One can consider two extremes of neurochemical transmission based upon the distance which the transmitter molecules must travel before acting upon a receptor.

Short-range synapses

At one extreme are the majority of synapses in the mammalian brain, where the pre- and post-synaptic membranes are in close proximity and the neurotransmitter has only a distance of a few micra (or even of Angstroms) to travel before reaching its receptor target. In most synapses of this type, there are enzymes present in the region of the synapse which can rapidly deactivate the neurotransmitter. Such synaptic contacts are well suited for the transmission and transformation of coded or pulsed information and can be considered to be analogous to the digital processing of information in computers. An example is the way in which the vertebrate nervous system progressively transforms spots of light striking the retina into line segments, edge detectors and eventually achieves complex pattern recognition. Pharmacological manipulations which alter the transmission patterns of such information processing systems can only produce disruptions of signal processing, such that the basic behaviours of the animal or the extent of physiological functioning will not be altered in some systematic, biased manner but will rather become erratic and disorganized. Many transmitters such as several amino acids, gamma-aminobutyric acid (GABA), and ACh appear likely to fall into this classification. The neurons, or cell bodies, of these neurotransmitters are present in many different brain regions. Pharmacological manipulations of such transmitters produce toxic-like, confused states in humans, such as that produced by the anti-cholinergic poisons present in several pesticides when they are accidentally ingested by agricultural workers. Comparisons of the roles of such neurotransmitters across species will be difficult, for other than cataloguing the amount and distribution of such transmitters in different species, and noting the evolution of new transmitters, it will be difficult to ascertain their basic functions in a comparative perspective.

Long-range chemical transmission

At the other extreme of chemical transmission lies long-range transmission, such as occurs with hormones. Here a chemical substance is released by a neurosecretory cell into the bloodstream, where it may travel anywhere within the body before reaching its target organ. Exact patterns of neural firing codes cannot play an important role in this type of long-range chemical transmission, and consequently pharmacological manipulations of such chemical substances produce biases in organized behaviour or physiologic function. Examples here are the fluctuations in complex, goal-directed behaviour produced by manipulations of gonadal hormones, or the widespread but physiologically consistent effects on body metabolism and brain activity produced by manipulations of thyroid secretions. Many such hormones have influences on the brain as well as on the body.

Cross-species comparison of these types of chemicals has been considerably more fruitful. For example, the central core, or medulla, of the adrenal gland secretes into the bloodstream two chemically related but distinct substances, epinephrine and norepinephrine. These two substances are both sympathomimetic (i.e. they both stimulate the peripheral sympathetic nervous system), but they do so in slightly different ways. Just as one can learn something about the recent life history of an animal by measuring the size of its adrenal gland (since chronic stress leads to an increase in the size of the adrenals due to their constant overactivity), one can also learn something about the ecological niche of that animal by comparing the ratio of epinephrine to norepinephrine. Mammals which are generally predators (such as the large members of the cat family) have more norepinephrine in their adrenals while animals which are predominantly hunted (such as rabbits) have a larger proportion of epinephrine. This ratio of norepinephrine to epinephrine is thought to vary somewhat in the urine of humans when the urine samples are taken following the viewing of an exciting film, such as a comedy, as opposed to viewing a frightening film. Here then is a case of two chemical substances which have some consistent relationship to functional behaviour which has retained a constancy of physiologic effects across a number of species.

Intermediate brain modulators of drive states

A variety of evidence implies that certain types of neurotransmitter systems present in the brain of vertebrates act somewhere between these two extremes. The monoamines dopamine, norepinephrine and serotonin are prime candidates for being intermediate neuromodulators of central drive states, emotion and mood. Some of the evidence for this is based on anatomical considerations.

The chief collections of cell bodies containing the monoamines lie in the brainstem, in and around the reticular formation (Figure 4.3). Brain lesion studies led early in the history of brain science to the conclusion that the neuronal circuitry within the brainstem core regions in and around the reticular formation developed as just such fundamental controllers of consciousness, attention and arousal. This control circuitry continued to develop projections to the higher regions of the brain as evolution progressed. Thus, inhibitory and facilitatory brainstem pathways were described where lesions or electrical stimulation would facilitate or inhibit lower spinal motor reflexes, spinal and brainstem sympathetic and parasympathetic reflexes, cardiovascular and respiratory centres, and equally well produce unresponsiveness and unconsciousness or, alternatively, enhanced responsivity and increased arousal in higher sensory, motor and integrative centres.

Massively branching cells from this region have been found to radiate out to innervate wide portions of the brain and to show long cycles of activity and inactivity, presumably reflecting the primitive brain's control over arousal. Norepinephrine-containing cells have been observed to branch diffusely, with the same cell sending axons to the cerebellum and to the visual cortex, two highly different brain regions. Such norepinephrine-containing cells appear poorly designed to carry discrete pieces of information (they branch too diffusely) but rather well designed to place the entire brain into different states of general arousal or emotion as demanded by the survival needs of the organism.

Considerable evidence from pharmacological experiments indicates that the monoamines exert important influences over general brain

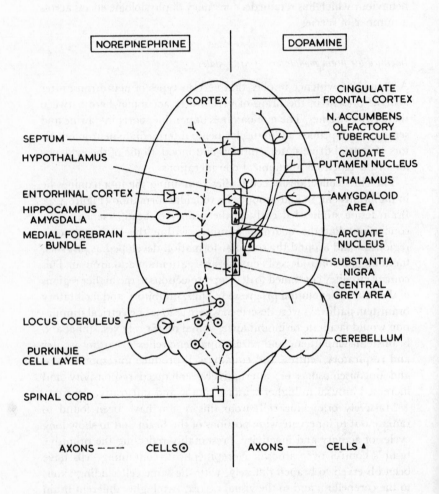

Fig. 4.3 Schematic representation of dopaminergic and noradrenergic pathways in the rat brain. Norepinephrine pathways and cell bodies are indicated on the left side of the illustration, while dopamine projections are shown on the right side. Figure adapted by Dr Stanley Watson from Lindvall and Bjorklund, and from Ungerstedt. From J. Barchas, P. Berger, R. Ciaranello and G. Elliot (eds). *Psychopharmacology: From Theory to Practice.* Copyright 1977, Oxford University Press.

function (Frankenhaeuser, 1971). A considerable array of evidence links the monoamines with the regulation of affect: in general, drugs which lower monoamine levels lower mood, and drugs which raise the levels of the monoamines raise mood. Drugs such as reserpine and tetrabenazine, which decrease the levels of the monoamines by preventing their storage, induce a psychological depression in some humans, and in monkeys and other mammals they induce a lethargic, withdrawn state characterized by irritability, weight loss, social withdrawal, decreased activity and other behaviours which seem to mimic those of human depressives. A common characteristic of a variety of pharmacological agents is that they all raise the levels of the monoamines at their synaptic targets: monoamine oxidase inhibitors doing so by partially preventing the breakdown of the monoamines, and tricyclic antidepressants doing so by blocking the reuptake of monoamines.' A wide variety of euphoriant and psychologically addicting drugs, such as the amphetamines, heroin and cocaine, have been shown to alter monoamine metabolism and alter the action of the monoamines at their receptive sites.

Other evidence from animal studies (Jouvet, 1972, for example) implicates these monoamines in the central modulation of a variety of emotional and other behaviours. Serotonin appears to be important for slow-wave sleep, in that animals depleted of serotonin through the use of synthesis inhibitors or discrete brain lesions become sleepless, as well as hyperaroused, hyperaggressive and hypersexual. Such animals also have lowered pain thresholds and, as sleep deprivation continues, become hallucinatory. Norepinephrine, conversely, appears to be more closely related to the production of arousal behaviours. Animals depleted of norepinephrine are less active than normals. Norepinephrine appears to be essential for aroused states such as rapid-eye-movement sleep, self-stimulation of the brain and feeding behaviour. Because there are too few actual norepinephrine and serotonin cell bodies to suggest that this widespread control over diverse brain functions could be very precise, it seems likely that these neurochemical systems are not intrinsically involved in the organization of emotional behaviours, but rather that they serve to regulate the appearance and timing of a large number of more specific neural circuits, such as those underlying species-specific behaviours. In other words, the monoamines appear to act to drive, energize or gate specifically organized cell assemblies as is appropriate for the survival of the organism. This would explain why the exact neuronal patterns of firing of monoamine cells do not seem essential for the organization of behaviour. Evidence for this conclusion is that when drugs which alter the patterns of monoamine cell firing (such as amphetamines or tranquillizers) are administered to humans, there is not a disorientation or clouding of consciousness nor are there indications of the toxic confusional states seen following other types of pharmacological agents. Instead, the human shows general alterations in alertness or arousal.

Norepinephrine-serotonin balance and behaviour

For a number of years I have studied the effects of alterations produced in monoamine systems on the behaviour of rats housed in isolation cages and tested in behavioural tasks, or in rats housed in enriched, semi-naturalistic rat colony environments. The results of these experiments (Ellison, 1975; 1977) are instructive in that they both indicate substantial differences between the behaviour of caged animals (as are usually studied in the laboratory) and those of animals in more naturalistic situations, and because they have led me to view the functions of central monoaminergic systems in terms of their evolutionary development.

Norepinephrine-depleted and serotonin-depleted animals behave oppositely on many tests. Norepinephrine-depleted animals have hunger deficits, underconsuming food, whereas serotonin-depleted animals consume more food than normals, do not increase their intake appreciably when deprived of food, and take their food in small, frequent meals. They behave as though constantly hungry, even when not deprived of food. When tested for avoidance of intense visual stimulation, norepinephrine-depleted animals become progressively more lethargic and inactive with continued testing whereas serotonin-depleted animals become progressively more agitated. The opposed behaviours of these two types of depleted animals can be seen best in open field tests. This involves removing an animal from its home cage, suddenly placing it in a novel environment consisting of a round enclosure, and recording the amount of locomotion, rearing up on the hindlegs, grooming and proportion of time spent in the centre of the enclosure as opposed to near the walls. Serotonin-depleted animals in this test appear to be frightened, hyperaroused animals: they stay near the walls of the enclosure, locomote less than normals because they 'freeze', and are hypervigilant in that they rear excessively. Norepinephrine-depleted animals behave oppositely: they blindly locomote all around the novel environment, entering the centre of the field even more than controls, but emit few rearing responses. These results imply that serotonin-depleted animals mimic aspects of human anxiety states, whereas norepinephrine-depleted animals mimic aspects of human depression and retardation. This conclusion is strengthened by the observation that those pharmacological agents which have been found effective in treating anxiety in humans predominantly are potentiators of serotonin, whereas those drugs used to treat fundamental depression are generally norepinephrine-potentiating agents.

When observed in semi-naturalistic rat colony environments, the behaviour of depleted animals is distinctively different but still in agreement with the above conclusion. Serotonin-depleted animals are hyperactive, remaining out of the burrows more than any other group and running in activity wheels the most. These animals also become progressively more hyperaggressive and competitive, especially during the hour of feeding. Norepinephrine-depleted animals tend to remain in the burrows more than any other group, and when out are inactive and tend to lose battles. Consequently they gradually fall to the bottom of the dominance hierarchy.

These observations have led me to think of these alterations in behaviour produced by monoamine neurotoxins in terms used by ethologists. The low-serotonin rat can be thought of as being in a state of central functioning appropriate for any animal out in the environment, foraging for food: it is hyperaroused, sensitive to stimulation and vigilant, and it is extremely frightened when confronted with a novel situation. The norepinephrine-depleted animal is conversely best thought of as in a state of functioning appropriate for an animal in his nest or burrow: underaroused and unresponsive to external stimulation, and thereby overconfident in the face of novelty.

The ergotropic-trophotropic dichotomy of Hess

These results suggest that the primitive neuronal systems from the midbrain which use as their neurotransmitters norepinephrine and serotonin perform functions stemming from early vertebrate evolution but that these systems have maintained control over the higher brain even in humans. The location of monoamine cell bodies deep in the brainstem suggests that these neuronal systems evolved initially at a level like that of the primitive aquatic vertebrate. Even at this primitive level, there is an extremely basic functional dichotomy between behaviours which expend energy (such as fight or flight) and those which conserve energy (such as rest). These two types of behaviours are related to a fundamental balance which all organisms must regulate: that between energy expenditure and energy conservation. For example, in order to replenish food reserves, an animal must venture from a place of rest or hiding into the environment, but this burns up energy. Energies expended during moments of stress must be replenished, and in fact energies must be stored away to stand ready for emergencies. There is a natural opposition between these two processes in the body – anabolism and catabolism – which develops into antagonistic emotional responses. To a certain extent, this dichotomy is related to the actions of the sympathetic nervous system (the spender of energies) and the parasympathetic nervous system (the accumulator of reserves). But the central innervations which develop to guide and control the behaviours essential for maintaining energy balance become related to different kinds of reinforcement or affectual control (Glickman and Schiff, 1967).

An aid to thinking about how these concepts relate to affect is a consideration of the different physical locations in which these two states occur. In most primitive animals there is some place or ecological niche where energy conservation occurs (rest, digestion, regeneration). This might be the school for a fish, the bird's nest, or the rat's burrow. Conversely, energy is expended out in the environment, but it is principally out in the environment that the consummatory responses biologically necessary for survival are made (such as predation and food seeking, exploration and territorial defence). When the primitive fish or terrestrial vertebrate was resting securely in its place of rest, one type of brain and body state was appropriate, and there are a huge number of physiological functions which would have adaptively been turned on, energized or allowed to operate. These functions comprise the trophotropic functions described by Hess (1964) and correspond to the low norepinephrine state previously described. As the organism leaves the nest this state of brain operation must be shut off and, when out meeting the environment, another and almost converse set of physiological and behavioural circuits are appropriate and should be energized (sympathetic dominance, arousal and vigilance high, approach and withdrawal systems activated and ready, etc.), corresponding to the ergotropic functions (i.e.

low serotonin). Furthermore, two antagonistic types of positive affect are suggested: one which pulled the primitive animal out of hiding and into the environment by positively rewarding him when he engaged in appetitive consummatory responses, but another which pulled him back into the security of the nest by satisfying a reciprocal set of needs. This emphasis on affects, or positively pulling forces, is implied by the words ergotropic (towards work or energy expenditure) and trophotropic (towards nourishment).

Table 4.2   Behaviour of rats in opposite states of monoamine imbalance and hypothesized locations and affectual correlates of these states

	State of monoamine imbalance	
Behaviour or correlate	Low serotonin High norepinephrine	Low norepinephrine High serotonin
Behaviour in familiar environment (observations in colony)	'Aroused and exploratory', in burrows less than controls, running in activity wheels, approach humans	'Driveless and withdrawn', stay in burrows, inactive, last to come to feeding
Behaviour in novel environment (open-field test)	'Frightened and paranoid', decreased locomotion (freezing), increased rearing (vigilant), stay near walls or hide under objects	'Fearless and nonvigilant', locomote more than controls, decreased rearing, enter centre of field, hide less than controls
Drug model	Amphetamines, stimulants	Heroin, barbiturates, tranquillizers
Physical location	Periphery of animal's territory	Centre of animal's territory
Positive affect	Excitement, approach towards goal objects	Security, relaxation
Negative affect	Anxiety, fear	Lack or arousal, depression
Hess's states	Ergotropic	Trophotropic

In Table 4.2 these considerations are summarized. The behaviour of animals placed in monoamine imbalance by injections of neurotoxins into the brain, or of injections of stimulant or depressant drugs, can be viewed as behaviour appropriate for an animal at either the periphery or the centre of his territory. Because this generalized scheme fits both behavioural and biochemical data derived from species as diverse as fish and mammals studied in the laboratory, on the one hand, and humans in the psychiatric clinic, on the other, it provides a framework on which more refined conceptualizations can be built. While the actual consummatory responses for satisfying basic needs in different animals are highly refined, consisting of species-specific behaviours, many of the most basic drives and biological rhythms are consistently present in very diverse species. The study of the neurochemical controllers of such basic functions, and thereby of the brain cells responsible for energizing or releasing such functions, may provide a method for uniquely studying evolution.

References

Blum, J., Kirshner, N. and Utley, J. (1966) The effect of reserpine on growth and catecholamine content of Tetrahymena. *Mol. Pharmacology 2*: 606–8.

Ellison, G. (1975) Behaviour and the balance between norepinephrine and serotonin. *Acta Neurobiol. Exp. 35*: 499–515.

Ellison, G. (1977) Animals models of psychopathology: the low-norepinephrine and low serotonin rat. *American Psychologist 32*: 1036–45.

Frankenhaeuser, M. (1971) Behaviour and circulating catecholamines. *Brain Research 31*: 241–62.

Glickman, S. and Schiff, B. (1967) A biological theory of reinforcement. *Psychological Review 74*: 81–109.

Hess, W. R. (1964) *The Biology of Mind*. Chicago: University of Chicago Press.

Iversen, S. D. and Iversen, L. L. (1975) Chemical pathways in the brain. In M. S. Gazzaniga and C. Blakemore (eds) *Handbook of Psychobiology*. London: Academic Press, 141–52.

Iversen, S. D., Iversen, L. L. and Snyder, S. (eds) (1975) Amino acid neurotransmitters. Vol. 4 of *Handbook of Psychopharmacology*. London: Plenum Press.

Jouvet, M. (1972) The role of monoamines and actylcholine-containing neurons in the regulation of the sleep-waking cycle. *Ergebnisse der physiol. 64*: 166–307.

Nielsen, M., Braestrup, C. and Squires, R. (1978) Evidence for a late evolutionary appearance of brain-specific benzodiazepine receptors: an investigation of 18 vertebrate and 5 invertebrate species. *Brain Research 141*: 342–6.

Welsh, J. and King, E. (1970) Catecholamines in Planaria. *Comparative Biochemistry and Physiology 36*: 683–8.

5 The evolution and function of sleep

Ray Meddis

Introduction

Recent scientific explorations of the nature and function of sleep have
concentrated on its electrophysiology. Whilst this has proved to be
an exciting and profitable exercise, this review will attempt a much
broader perspective by acknowledging at least three quite different
aspects of sleep: experience, behaviour and physiology. After all, sleep
is not only found in the physiology laboratory: it is something which
we all experience regularly and something which we see other people
and other animals doing every day. We look to science for a better
understanding of why we do it and what happens while we are doing
it and therefore the success of the scientific endeavour must be judged
by the light it throws on our everyday experience of a very common
phenomenon. In particular, sleep appears to have a long evolutionary
history and one of the purposes of this chapter is to show how a comparative, developmental and evolutionary study of sleep may assist
in our understanding of its presence in man.

It is tempting to imagine that sleep is a blank period, a time of
no experience, but this is an illusion of memory. When we wake
sleeping people and gently but firmly probe their immediate recall
of what they were thinking about, we find nearly always that something was going on but the memory slips away at tantalizing speed.

Sleepers may not admit they were asleep but insist that they were merely lying thinking. They may report thought sequences drifting loosely from one topic to another or obsessively repeating themselves. At another time they narrate vivid dream sequences full of interest and action. More rarely one gets a nightmare report full of menacing images and a sense of overwhelming helplessness and paralysis. While falling asleep, people may hallucinate loud bangs, or the sound of a person calling one's name – the so called 'hypnopompic' phenomena. There is no truth to the notion that the mind rests during sleep; it continues to be very active. Only the memory for sleep experience is deficient even for night terrors which may involve screaming and clambering out of bed (Oswald, 1974, p. 100). An experience may be caught if the individual is woken at the time but, if we wait till morning, all is usually lost.

Mental activity during sleep is halfway between the reasonable and bizarre. We think and dream of people, places, things and events we know and recognize but these occur in odd and often unreasonable combinations and sequences to generate tantalizing narratives which, like the ramblings of schizophrenia, continually appear to verge on the meaningful and significant. Undoubtedly, the fascination of all civilized peoples with the meaning of dreams must be largely attributed to the incomplete coherence of the dream narrative but for some the pursuit of significance in dreams has been seen as enormously profitable (Cartwright, 1977). Biology cannot as yet illuminate the significance of dreams; but see Dement (1972, ch. 4), Webb (1975, ch. 13), Oswald (1974, ch. 4) for a variety of opinions.

Sleep-related experiences do not occur only while we are asleep but begin long before and persist long after the sleep period. Drowsiness is the most obvious phenomenon. It occurs prior to sleep (where it may facilitate sleep onset) and on waking. Phenomenologically, it consists of a gradual lowering of awareness and interest in one's surroundings along with an increasing reluctance to engage in any task requiring effort or attention. Drowsiness can be banished rapidly if an external stimulus carries enough urgency, but the more drowsy we are, the more urgent the stimulus needs to be. Drowsiness and the desire for sleep extend the domain of sleep-related phenomena far into the worlds of wakefulness.

To analyse sleep from a behavioural point of view may also seem rather pointless, since sleep is a period when animals and men appear to be doing nothing at all. However, the suppression of action can itself be a significant way of controlling behaviour, as it is in passive avoidance, freezing in the presence of predators or reducing mobility in preparation for hibernation. We assume that the immobility of sleep is engineered for a purpose, but what purpose? Is it an avoidance response which hides an animal away from predators, conserves energy and isolates the animal from the inclemencies of the environment – like hibernation? Or is it a period of rest following fatigue when physiological and psychological recovery can take place? This is the unsolved problem of the function of sleep to which we must return later.

'Doing nothing' is a carefully organized business when it comes to sleep. It occurs almost invariably in a species-specific site, which is carefully chosen according to the needs of the particular type of animal, and in some cases a nest or lair may be specially constructed for the purpose. The sleeping animal adopts a characteristic sleep posture which is again carefully chosen to suit the prevailing environmental conditions. The timing of sleep is commonly regulated by an internal twenty-four hour clock which, while partly independent of the day-night (or tidal) cycle, is usually synchronized with it. The result is that sleep usually occurs at a particular time within the twenty-four hour cycle, whenever is best suited to the animal's needs. The sleep period is characterized not by an unconscious coma-like state, but merely by raised response thresholds. Thus a sleeping animal behaves as if it is continually monitoring its environment but chooses to respond only if the matter is very urgent. Finally, an animal makes strenuous efforts to get into a situation where it can fall asleep and will overcome serious obstacles to do so. If woken from sleep, this 'sleep drive' initiates further efforts to get back to sleep as soon as possible. These five factors combined have led at least one ethologist (Tinbergen, 1951, p. 106) to view sleep not merely as a state of inactivity but as a motivated sequence of carefully tailored behaviours culminating in a prolonged period of immobility.

The most impressive recent advances have, however, come from electrophysiological studies where measures of EEG activity, heart rate, respiration rate, eye movements and muscle tonus have shown important correlations with sleep behaviour. Unfortunately, the patterns recorded are quite complex and not easily described quickly. The problem is that the electrophysiological indicators show not one sleep state but many, and the number of states which can be found vary between animal species. A routine classification system for man

(Rechtschaffen and Kales, 1968) specifies a minimum of five, whereas, for rats, most researchers restrict themselves to two sleep states, and among reptiles no one has made a convincing case for their being more than one identifiable state.

Among warm-blooded animals (birds and mammals) it is common to distinguish two broad categories of sleep states: quiet sleep (QS) and active sleep (AS). QS is characterized by high voltage slow wave (less than 2 Hz) activity in the EEG trace. This has earned it the alternative (but confusing) name of slow wave sleep. In most mammals (but not birds), these slow waves are accompanied by brief bursts (1–2 sec) of faster (12 Hz) waves called 'spindles'. Cats and all primates so far tested show two types of QS known as deep quiet sleep (DQS) and light quiet sleep (LQS). DQS is dominated by high voltage slow wave EEG activity, while LQS has fewer slow waves but continues to show spindling. In man, QS is divided into four substages according to how much slow wave activity is present. Stage 4, for example, is dominated by slow waves, while stage 2 has very little and is diagnosed mainly from the presence of spindles and a new wave form, the 'K-complex', which appears at irregular intervals. This appears on the EEG trace as a single negative/positive swing with a return to baseline lasting a second or two. Stage 1 has no slow wave activity at all and occurs mainly as the individual is falling asleep. This is accompanied by slow rolling (side-to-side) movements of the eyes. Unfortunately, we do not understand the significance of spindles, k-complexes, or even slow waves, and they are at present merely used to help us classify the different stages. Examples of these types of EEG record are given later in Figure 5.3.

The second major sleep state category is active sleep (AS), which alternates slowly with QS through the sleep period and is characterized by a flat EEG trace similar to a waking EEG pattern. In birds and mammals this state is also characterized by episodes of rapid eye movements (REMs) which gave rise to the earlier name of REM sleep. This name is unfortunate, since REMs are only one of many symptoms of AS. Other symptoms include twitching of the extremities (fingers, paws, lips, whiskers), irregular heart and breathing rate, a particularly deep relaxation of the main postural muscles, continuous 6 Hz electrical activity in the hippocampus, electrical 'spike' activity in the pons (PGO spikes), and – most curious of all – penile erections in man. All this is in sharp contrast to the uneventful physiology of QS. It is not surprising that this state earned the name of paradoxical sleep when it was first discovered. Also, the most vivid dreaming reports are obtained when sleeping subjects are woken from this particular stage.

It is common to view the symptoms of AS as a result of the superimposed action of two separate systems known as tonic and phasic. The phasic component is presumed to be responsible for the twitching of the extremities, eye movements, PGO spikes, irregularities of heartbeat and breathing as well as bursts of 7–12 Hz activity in the hippocampus. The tonic component is presumed responsible for the steady EEG pattern, the steady 6 Hz electrical waveform in the hippocampus, the persisting reduction in postural muscle tonus and penile erections. Under certain conditions, including the administration of certain drugs such as atropine sulphate and ether anaesthesia, it is possible to knock out one of these systems, selectively leaving the other operating normally (Robinson et al., 1977). Nevertheless, for most purposes, analysis of sleep records usually involves simply scoring the presence or absence of AS.

The discovery of the two major types of sleep is still quite recent and much of this article will be concerned with the problems of deciding what significance to attach to their existence. Although there is no shortage of theories, so far there is little consensus as to why sleep should be so complicated. There is no doubt that these developments are very important but our ignorance at all points remains profound. The reader should therefore consider the facts which follow as little more than clues to an unsolved riddle.

Moreover, we must not adopt too simplistic a view of the relationship between sleep and its electrophysiological correlates. It is true that the electrophysiological signs and symptoms discussed above do occur when the individual is asleep. This does not mean that the correlation is perfect. It is not uncommon to find a disagreement between the individual's own impressions and the judgement of the EEG machine. For example Webb (1975, p. 14) woke people forty-five minutes after they had been left alone to go to sleep and asked them if they had, in fact fallen asleep. Of those who had reached the deepest stages (3 and 4) of QS, 10 per cent said that they had not. Of those who reached only stage 1, 60 per cent said that they had not. If we knew more than we do about the significance of spindles, k-complexes and slow wave electrical activity, we might be able to resolve these discrepancies. For the present, we must simply accept that sleep, as a behavioural, phenomenological and electrophysiological affair, is still only a moderately coherent concept. The question 'What is sleep?' remains fairly open.

Comparative study of sleep

One obvious way of extending our understanding is to study sleep in species other than ourselves. Of course, in doing so we must restrict ourselves to behavioural and electrophysiological studies, but the information gathered in this way has proved so surprising and challenging that the effort has been well worthwhile. Sleep, it seems, is very much more more widespread in the animal kingdom than we generally recognize, that is, if we agree to use the behavioural criteria given earlier. These involve periods of prolonged immobility, with raised response thresholds, which take place in a species-specific sleep site with a species-specific sleep posture and which are organized according to a circadian (or tidal) cycle. Not all of these conditions are met in each animal, but there are usually enough to make the presence of sleep reasonably unambiguous to even the untrained observer. In this way we can show that sleep can be found among mammals, birds, reptiles, amphibia, fish and even molluscs and insects (Meddis, 1977, ch. 2).

The electrophysiological measures do not show the same continuity across types of animals. EEG techniques show reasonable similarities among mammals and birds but such sleep signs as high voltage slow waves are not a regular feature of sleep in reptiles, amphibia, fish, molluscs and insects. This is partly because different types of animals have important differences in brain structure – for example, reptiles do not show the same development of the cortex where many of the crucial electrophysiological signs are found. Electrophysiology is not yet up to the job of diagnosing sleep in reptiles, and we are forced to rely on behavioural evidence when discussing sleep in species other than mammals and birds.

For the moment, let us restrict our attention to studies of mammals, where a fascinating picture has been revealed by electrophysiological studies. Figure 5.1 shows roughly how much AS and QS are taken by various species studied mainly in the laboratory. To find the total time spent sleeping every day by a given species simply add the time spent in QS to the time spent in AS. Thus the North American opossum spends 19·4 hours (13·8 + 5·6) in total sleep time (TST) while the horse enjoys only 2·9 (2·1 + 0·8) in total. This is an interesting

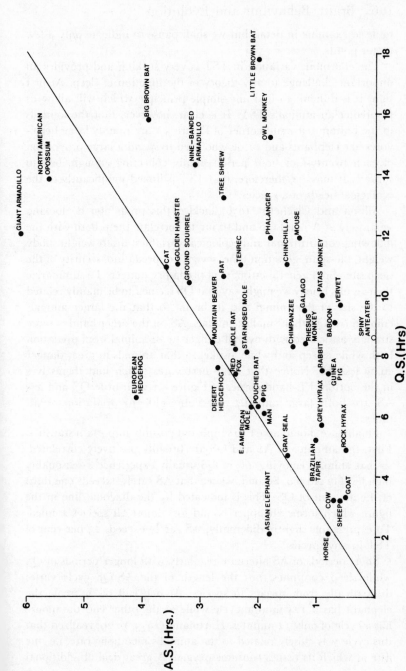

Fig. 5.1   Estimates of hours per day spend in quiet sleep (QS) and active sleep (AS). Data supplied by T. Allison, Yale University, s used in Allison and Cicchetti (1976). References to studies of individual animals are given in Meddis (1975).

table to examine in detail but we shall pause to indicate only a few major points.

The enormous variation in TST is very striking and provides an important challenge to any theory of the function of sleep. At first sight it is difficult to find any simple principle which will allow us to predict an animal's TST. It is clear, however, that the animals in the bottom left-hand corner of Figure 5.1 are mainly large herbivores like elephants and cattle who need to spend a large proportion of each twenty-four hour period simply collecting enough food to survive. It may be, therefore, that TST is linked significantly to the ecological needs of a species.

Allison and Cicchetti (1976) tackled this prediction by looking separately at AS and QS and trying to correlate them both with the following constitutional and ecological variables: brain weight, body weight, life-span, gestation time, severity of predation, security of the sleep site and a general estimate of predatory danger. To summarize their results briefly we might say that QS seemed to be mainly related to the size of the animal and its brain, so that the larger animals enjoyed *less* QS than smaller animals. AS on the other hand is more strongly associated with overall danger to an animal from predation both while asleep and while awake, so that animals in great danger enjoy less AS. Notice that large herbivores which find themselves in the bottom left-hand corner of Figure 5.1 with little QS and less AS are both large animals and vulnerable to predation at all times.

Finally, we should note two simple but possibly important statistics. First, the amounts of AS and QS are broadly positively correlated, so that animals enjoying lots of QS usually experience a reasonably high level of AS too. Second, we see that AS rarely exceeds one third of the amount of QS. This is indicated by the diagonal line in the figure which forms an upper bound for almost all species studied. To express this slightly differently, AS rarely exceeds 25 per cent of TST in any species.

Short periods of AS alternate regularly with longer periods of QS while sleep continues, but the length of the AS/QS cycle varies dramatically from species to species. At one end of the scale the elephant has a 124 minute cycle while at the other end the mouse has a cycle of only 12 minutes. Hartmann (1973, p. 29) realized that this cycle was closely related to the animal's metabolic rate, i.e. the rate at which its tissues consume oxygen. A great deal of additional

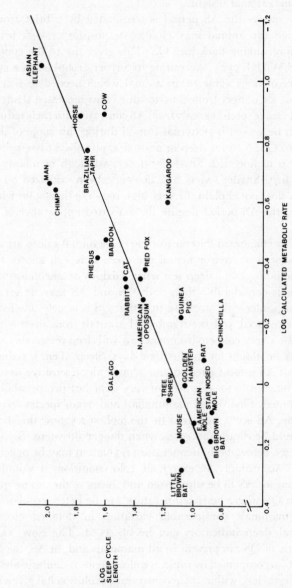

Fig. 5.2 Relationship of metabolic rate to duration of QS/AS sleep cycle length. See Figure 5.1 for notes on data used.

evidence has since become available (Figure 5.2) which has amply confirmed his original insight.

In many species the AS period is terminated by a brief arousal during which the animal may change its posture or look briefly around before sinking back into QS. This gives rise to the concept of a QS/AS/WAKE cycle. According to Snyder (1966), such a cycle would be of obvious value to an animal which needed to scan its environment for danger from time to time. This increased tendency of animals to wake spontaneously from AS contrasts with their reduced tendency to be woken by external stimuli during this stage of sleep compared to QS. Natural sleep in normal adults always begins with QS, which is in line with Snyder's theory, although in infants AS may come first. Snyder's view has, however, been criticized on the basis that it does not explain the very high response thresholds which exist during the AS period despite the activated appearance of the EEG.

Day-to-day changes in the constitution of an animal's sleep are also carefully tailored to environmental pressures. It is well known that animals, including man, sleep less when anxious or uncomfortable. If the stress is considerable then both QS and AS may be greatly reduced, but under mild stress we find that QS is largely unaffected while AS is reduced and the number of arousals from sleep is also increased. In a very cold environment cats will sleep reasonably well but AS may be absent for the first few days. Sleep, then, is reduced by stress, but AS is most affected and is often alone sensitive to mild stressors. The reasons for this are not very clear but two possibilities should be noted. First, in all mammalian and avian species, except possibly man, AS is characterized by the highest response thresholds and this could be disadvantageous when danger threatens. Second, as we shall see below, body temperature regulation may be deficient during AS. Accordingly, in extremely cold conditions it would be advantageous for AS to be suppressed and for more time to be spent awake or in QS where body temperature can be better regulated.

Among mammals considerable variation in detailed electro-physiological sleep indicators can be observed. The slow waves characteristic of QS are present in all mammals and, in AS, the low voltage EEG accompanied by rapid eye movements is similarly always visible. Nevertheless, within these constraints, evolution has given rise to considerable variation among the detailed indicators such as the presence or absence of k-complexes and spindles. Figure 5.3 looks at some important features of sleep in man in terms of their presence or absence in other mammals, in birds and in reptiles. The arrows to the left of this figure represent major lines of vertebrate evolution. The specific ordering of animals in the body of the figure, however, is based on the number of sleep features which modern representatives of each animal form display, and this suggests the following phylogenetic sequence of additions: slow waves, spindles, light/deep QS distinction, k-complexes. At the bottom of Figure 5.3 is given the approximate age at which these signs appear in the human neonate.

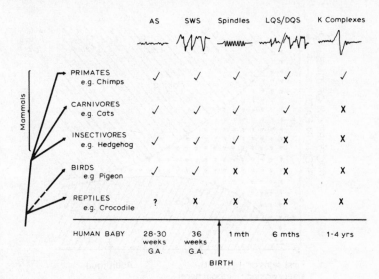

	AS	SWS	Spindles	LQS/DQS	K Complexes
PRIMATES e.g. Chimps	✓	✓	✓	✓	✓
CARNIVORES e.g. Cats	✓	✓	✓	✓	X
INSECTIVORES e.g. Hedgehog	✓	✓	✓	X	X
BIRDS e.g. Pigeon	✓	✓	X	X	X
REPTILES e.g. Crocodile	?	X	X	X	X
HUMAN BABY	28-30 weeks G.A.	36 weeks G.A.	1 mth	6 mths	1-4 yrs

Mammals

BIRTH

Fig. 5.3   Phylogeny of EEG sleep indicators. LQS = light quiet sleep; DQS = deep quiet sleep; SWS = slow wave sleep; AS = active sleep; G.A = gestation age.

It can be seen that the ontogenetic and phylogenetic patterns mirror each other very well. Once again, it is difficult to know what significance can be attached to these facts since we do not understand the function of the EEG indicators but we shall use the correlation between ontogeny and phylogeny later when speculating about the evolution of the AS/QS cycle.

Ontogeny

The accumulation of many studies allows us to draw a number of

firm conclusions about the development of sleep patterns from birth
to old age. First, we know from studies of the premature infant and
animal foetus that electrophysiological sleep signs appear before birth.
Second, we know that infants sleep longer than adults and that the
proportion of AS also is considerably greater at this time. For example,
at birth, a human infant sleeps for approximately sixteen hours on
average, but spends up to half of this time in AS (or more if it is
born prematurely). An infant kitten sleeps for almost the whole day

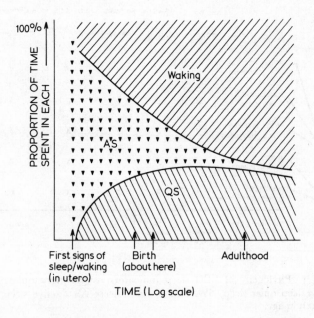

Fig. 5.4   General scheme of ontogeny of sleep states in mammals.

and almost all of this is spent in AS. Figure 5.4 summarizes the changes
which take place in all mammals studied so far between the appearance of the first signs of sleep through to adulthood. The percentages
vary from species to species, as does the actual point of birth in the
sequence, but the general pattern of development remains the same.
In human infants, sleep is distributed somewhat erratically across the
twenty-four hour period and occurs for much shorter periods on
average. The consolidation of sleep into one long period at night
occurs fairly quickly during the first month but naps in the morning

and afternoon may persist for two to four years (Webb, 1975, ch. 4).

Physiology

Although energy consumption during sleep is considerably lower than during active wakefulness, it is only slightly (10 per cent) lower than during relaxed wakefulness. In man, energy consumption is at its lowest during DQS when responsiveness is least and body movements are minimal. Muscle tension can however remain moderately high during QS and it is only during AS that the main postural muscles show any signs of deep relaxation. Because sleep typically occurs during the trough of the circadian rhythm (when body temperature, muscle tonus and energy consumption are very low), it is often difficult to decide to what degree the reduction in energy consumption during sleep can be ascribed to sleep *per se* or simply to the time of day, the reduction in body movements, lower body temperature and the existence of bed clothes to keep the sleeper warm.

At least four different hormones are known to show elevated levels of concentration in the blood during sleep: growth hormone (GH), prolactin, luteinizing hormone and testosterone (Adams and Oswald, 1977). Experiments have shown that some of the changes in hormone concentration are actually triggered by the presence of sleep, and not simply features of the circadian rhythm or a rebound effect following cessation of activity. The greatest experimental effort has been expended on GH release which is known to be triggered by DQS in man and baboons but not in dogs, cats, rats or rhesus monkeys. Some uncertainty surrounds the evaluation of the significance of the DQS related peak in GH release. This might indicate, on the one hand, an increased rate of protein molecule building or, alternatively, a period during which protein molecule breakdown is spared by providing an alternative route for the generation of energy through fat mobilization. A final decision on this issue may be delayed since the animals most suitable for the study of protein synthesis (cats, rats, hamsters) do not show the sleep-dependent GH release pattern. However, one study from the USSR (quoted by Adams and Oswald, 1977) indicated that the protein and RNA content of cells in the supra-optic nuclei of the brain is higher for sleeping rats than for waking rats.

AS, which in the adult occupies less than 25 per cent of the sleep period, has produced a long list of surprising physiological features. We already know that during AS the eyes are given to move rapidly to and fro in bursts which are correlated with twitching of fingers, toes, paws, whiskers, tail, etc. Whilst the muscles at the extremities are obviously active, the main postural muscles often show a profound loss of muscle tonus which explains the floppy supine posture of most mammals at this time. Heartbeat and respiration are variable even though the *average* values for heart and respiration rate may not differ greatly from QS levels. Blood pressure is moderately raised and less regular. The penis is commonly erect in men. The distribution of blood supply appears to change as blood flow to the periphery (and the musculature) is reduced while blood flow to the brain is increased. The full significance of these changes is unclear but Oswald (1974, p. 148) notes that the heat output of the brain rises at the same time as these blood flow changes. Recent evidence has shown that normal thermoregulating responses seem to be inactive during AS even though they occur normally during QS. Evidence of a failure of a variety of related mechanisms is available for a number of species including man (reducing sweating), cat (failure to shiver or pant), kangaroo rat (failure to raise metabolic rate in cold conditions), and cow (failure of nasolabial secretions). How do animals survive extremes of temperature if they fail to thermoregulate during AS? Fortunately, most animals' AS periods are short and, if body temperature falls too low, the animal responds by waking up. If the cold (or extreme heat) persists, AS is also either suppressed or greatly reduced. It is significant that the kangaroo rat when entering hibernation appears to suppress AS almost entirely; presumably because, at this time, delicate control of body temperature is essential.

Whilst it is tempting to concentrate narrowly on temperature regulation, we must pause to acknowledge the anomalous physiological activity in other spheres. During AS adrenalin flow may be considerably elevated (Oswald, 1974, p. 77) and this may be responsible for some of the cardiovascular changes noted. This rise in adrenalin concentration is associated with more fearful dreams but it is difficult to say which is cause and which effect. Nevertheless, such unregulated changes with no obvious purpose can be harmful and are thought to be responsible for many of the attacks of heart pain which occur at night and which typically occur during AS. Acid secretion in the stomach is also known to be raised during AS for stomach ulcer patients, and this is thought to be responsible for their painful awakenings at night. In cattle, all aspects of rumination cease abruptly when AS begins. Irregularities in the respiration of newborn human infants in the form of apneic (cessation of breathing) episodes lasting often longer than 10 secs are known to occur during sleep and they are up to six times more likely to occur during AS. If, as some believe, these apneic episodes may be involved in the sudden infant death syndrome (cot death), AS is clearly a period of increased vulnerability. All of these observations contribute to a picture of AS as a very unfamiliar and potentially dangerous physiological state.

Neuroanatomy

It is almost certainly true that every brain structure is affected by the transition from waking to sleep and from one sleep state to another. However, some parts of the brain are more affected by the state change than instrumental in causing it. For example, we can still observe sleeping and waking patterns of behaviour in rats even when the cerebral cortex has been removed. During their sleep episodes we can detect the alternation of QS and AS even though we can obviously not measure the high voltage slow wave activity during QS. What happens is that the AS state is readily diagnosed from the drop in muscle tonus, twitching at the extremities, rapid eye movement, hippocampal theta rhythm, etc. Between these AS episodes, however, the animal remains behaviourally asleep in a manner consistent with descriptions of QS. Thus, sleep is quite possible even in the absence of a cortex. Nevertheless, it would be foolish to infer that under normal circumstances the cortex did not play a role in regulating sleep both by helping and delaying the onset of sleep according to the current circumstances, as well as by interrupting sleep following stimuli of high motivational significance.

With this caution in mind, we may briefly consider a number of structures which have received intensive investigation in recent years and which may prove to be of central importance in understanding the sleep control mechanisms in animals. These are the midbrain reticular formation, the raphé nuclei, the nuclei locus coeruleus and subcoeruleus and the hippocampus (see Chapter 2 this volume). For two important reasons it is impossible to provide a satisfactory account of the results of this research. First, so much of it is recent that no universally accepted interpretation of the results has yet emerged and, second, the matter is so complex and in need of detailed qualification that I can no more than offer a flavour of what is happening in a few paragraphs.

The reticular formation has long been known to play an important role in the maintenance of wakefulness, since lesions in this area typically result in a comatose animal. Studies of various types have contributed to an overall picture of the reticular formation as a system which arouses and facilitates neural activity in both higher (e.g. cortical) and lower (e.g. spinal) structures through a very diffuse set of nerves radiating to all areas of the brain. The activity of this system is itself influenced by activity elsewhere in the brain which may either stimulate or suppress reticular formation activity.

Nearby, the raphé nuclei have been strongly implicated in the specific control of sleep onset and maintenance. These nuclei are rich in the neurotransmitter serotonin (see Chapter 4 of this volume) and have axons which travel to many parts of the brain, branching many hundreds of times on the way. When these cells are surgically destroyed or when the serotonin is depleted biochemically, severe insomnia ensues.

Close to the raphé nuclei lie the nucleus locus coeruleus and subcoeruleus, which are rich in noradrenalin (norepinephrine), a quite different neurotransmitter. Like the raphé nuclei, these too have a diffuse ascending and descending set of axons with a wide sphere of influence. Experiments have shown that they may be involved in the control of AS by interacting in some, as yet unclear, way with the raphé nuclei. Certainly the locus coeruleus is involved in the descending inhibition of motor activity which is responsible for the very low muscle tonus during AS. These nerve centres have also been implicated in important waking functions such as aggression and learning, so we must avoid too simplistic a view of their function.

Recent research into the functioning of the hippocampus has shown some interesting parallels with AS phenomena. We mentioned above that AS has both tonic and phasic aspects. The tonic aspects (e.g. cortical activation and low postural muscle tonus) are accompanied by continuous 6 Hz sinusoidal activity in the hippocampus while the phasic aspects (e.g. muscle twitches) are accompanied by brief bursts of 7–12 Hz activity also in the hippocampus. The phasic aspects could be suppressed leaving the tonic aspects intact using the drug Urethene while the opposite effect could be achieved using atropine sulphate (Robinson et al., 1977). The electrical activity of the hippocampus is also correlated with motor activity during wakefulness and is known to be influenced by ascending connections from the nucleus locus coeruleus. We may expect that future research into these structures will yield important insights into the neurological control of both sleep and waking.

Evolution of sleep

Sleep, when viewed behaviourally, is obviously very ancient and its origins will probably be hard to find. Certainly, among vertebrates, sleep behaviour is very common indeed. The basic features of immobility, specific sleep sites and postures and circadian organization are pretty much the same from one species to another despite some variation in the pattern of electrophysiological signs. The QS/AS cycle, however, shows a dramatic phylogenetic discontinuity which deserves our attention. Reptiles do not show any obvious cycle of this kind during sleep. This is surprising since both birds and mammals do show it even though they are thought to have evolved independently from reptilian ancestors (see Introduction to this volume, Figure 1). It has been suggested by Allison (1970) that the dividing line seems to lie between poikilotherms (cold-blooded animals) and homeotherms (warm-blooded animals). This seems to be a pretty adequate rule except for a single case (discovered by Allison himself) of the primitive egg-laying mammal, the spiny anteater, which shows no AS.

If reptiles, amphibia and fish show sleep but no regular alternation of two major sleep states, then it becomes reasonable to ask whether their sleep is QS or AS. There is no logical necessity that it should be either, but it is tempting to assume that homeotherms inherited one type of sleep from poikilotherms and invented a second for their own purposes. The generally accepted view among sleep researchers is that reptile sleep corresponds to QS in mammals and birds. The reasons for this view are mainly that sleep in fish and reptiles demonstrates few of the signs of agitation which characterize AS in homeotherms. If reptile sleep were continuous AS, we might expect to see a great many rapid eye movements, twitching of the extremities, irregularities of heart and respiration rates; but we do not. Moreover, Allison's failure to observe these symptoms in the mammalian spiny anteater further supports the view that AS is a relatively new invention, although it leaves some mystery surrounding the parallel evolution of AS in birds.

I have disagreed with this view for some time and my reasons for doing so are given in detail elsewhere (Meddis, 1977, ch. 6). However, I shall summarize my argument here because the evolutionary scheme which emerges provides an important alternative perspective when it comes to evaluating the possible functions of sleep.

To begin, it is important to discount the idea that reptiles ought to show continuous rapid eye movements, twitches and irregularities of physiological functioning if their sleep were the forerunner of AS in homeotherms. On the contrary, we may expect some phasic phenomena but these will be widely spaced and unimpressive because of the greatly reduced level of metabolic activity to be found in reptiles. Sleeping reptiles allow their body temperature to fall so that their low levels of metabolic activity are reduced even further and phasic events should become even more widely spaced and have lower amplitude. In fact, some reptiles and fish do show occasional phasic phenomena such as eye movements just as we might expect, but these are much rarer and more widely spaced in time than among mammals. We should also note that the reptilian EEG does not, as a rule, show high voltage slow waves but shows only a small increase in amplitude and slowing of rhythm of the waking EEG – a finding which is more consistent with a diagnosis of AS. Similarly, muscle tonus disappears completely during prolonged sleep in reptiles. This is also observed to be the case in avian and mammalian AS.

I do not believe, however, that the case for or against the idea of a reptilian origin of AS can be decided on this kind of evidence alone. Fortunately, there is much more evidence, for example the pattern of ontogenetic development, whereby AS can be observed in the mammalian foetus *before* QS. This might be taken as an indicator that AS preceded QS in phylogeny (using the rule 'ontogency recapitulates phylogeny'). Sleep researchers were aware of this possibility but have rejected it on the grounds that reptile sleep seemed so different from mammalian or avian AS. Since then, more evidence has emerged to allow us to assess the credibility of the ontogeny argument. In Figure 5.3 we see that the sequence of the development of various EEG indicators such as high voltage slow waves, spindles, the distinction between LQS and DQS and k-complexes, follows the possible sequence of phylogenetic development. If the rule that ontogeny recapitulates phylogeny applies to this aspect of the EEG of sleep, then we might expect that it applies equally well to the emergence of AS.

Exceptions to this rule do occur if a particular mechanism evolves late to serve a particular role in foetal development. Roffwarg et al. (1966) have suggested just such a theory, which implies that the foetus needs extra brain stimulation which is supplied by the excitement of AS. If they could prove that such a need exists, and that AS satisfies this need, then the theory could be very strong indeed, since AS proportions drop dramatically after infancy. However, it is not clear that such a need does exist nor that AS provides more neural stimulation than wakefulness in the foetus. We must therefore be cautious before concluding that AS evolved particularly to meet a need in the mammalian foetus.

Let us consider another pair of clues which we have met. First, the AS/QS cycle is only observed in homeotherms, i.e. animals who regulate their body temperatures using physiological means. Second, during AS in mammals, temperature regulation does not seem to function properly. It is therefore possible that AS is a primitive kind of sleep inherited from reptiles which do not attempt to regulate their body temperature during sleep. Failure to thermoregulate for long periods in homeotherms is a serious and ultimately fatal issue. However, thermoregulation functions effectively during QS and this prompts the idea that QS evolved later to rescue the poor homeotherm from a difficult situation. If this is true, we have a ready explanation of why AS and QS take turns – to prevent long periods of AS. It also explains why the proportion of sleep given over to AS drops dramatically after birth – because at this time the infant becomes responsible for maintaining his own body temperature. Small animals whose body temperature is most rapidly affected by environmental heat or cold are most threatened by AS. This explains the function shown in Figure 5.2 where animals with a low body weight (and therefore high metabolic rate) have a faster cycle time, because a faster cycle automatically reduces the duration of each AS episode.

The total argument is more general than this and involves other aspects of AS which are disadvantageous to warm-blooded animals but do not necessarily affect reptiles, amphibia or fish. These include high response thresholds in sleep, apneic episodes in infants and failure of rumination. If my view is correct, then we might reasonably expect even more surprises from future studies of the physiology of AS, since the theory predicts that failures of characteristically mammalian physiological mechanisms should be very common. If this expectation is confirmed,* it will help to establish the currently unpopular view that AS is phylogenetically older than QS and that the evolution of QS is to be understood in terms of the need for an alternative quiescent state which was more nicely tailored to the needs of homeotherms.

Sleep deprivation

One of the most significant aspects of sleep is that people resist being deprived of it. Prolonged sleep-loss always leads to increased sleepiness and a reduced interest in doing anything other than sleeping. This manifests itself in the form of impaired concentration and consequently increased errors in any task which we force ourselves to attempt. We can readily explain this in terms of a mechanism which uses drowsiness as a means to oblige animals to spend a proportion of their life in 'low profile' immobility (sleep). But is there a special sleep-deprivation condition which results directly from the lack of an important recovery process which would normally occur during sleep? If there is, then this deficit will point the way to understanding the function of sleep. Therein lay the importance of sleep deprivation studies to many sleep researchers who saw this as an important practical and theoretical problem.

Because sleep contains at least two major states, QS and AS, and because, in man, QS is divisible easily into substates, LQS (stages 1 and 2) and DQS (stages 3 and 4), sleep deprivation studies have become very complicated. We can either totally deprive a person of sleep or partially deprive him of AS or QS or DQS. (Attempts selectively to deprive persons of LQS are usually unsuccessful because that person is usually prevented from getting any sleep at all!) It will therefore prove difficult to summarize the results. However, most sleep researchers would agree that these studies have not taken us very far towards identifying any physiological deficit which could unambiguously be attributed to the loss of specific sleep recovery processes. The reader will need to check this generalization against his own reading in this area, e.g. Webb (1975), Dement (1972) and Oswald (1974). For the present, I shall confine my attention to a number of important points.

Sleep deprivation usually, but not always, results in a rebound increase in whatever was deprived when normal sleep conditions are resumed. Thus deprivation of AS or DQS leads to a rebound increase above normal levels on a recovery night and common experience suggests that a similar effect follows total sleep deprivation. However, some qualifications to this generalization are necessary. First, not all persons show this rebound, and some people recover without departing significantly from their normal sleep profile. Second, the rebound increase is usually only a fraction of what is lost and the more that is lost the smaller is the fraction recovered. No serious attempt is made to recover all of the lost sleep time.

There are two very different ways of explaining this rebound phenomenon. The most popular approach is to assume that the lack of sleep (QS, AS or both) causes some physiological deficit which in turn causes an increase in the pressure to sleep. This is a homeostatic theory with similarities to current views of hunger motivation. An alternative approach is to class the sleep drive with non-homeostatic drives such as sex or curiosity which also show a rebound phenomenon after periods during which outlets for the drive have been blocked. Rats, for example, will spend much longer in their running wheel than usual if their access to it is denied for a few days. In this case, we are dealing with a mechanism whose function appears to be to regulate, according to some general plan, the proportion of time an animal spends in different activities. If an opportunity to carry out a given activity is denied at one time, then later, when the situation permits, more time is set aside for this activity. It is not yet clear how we can decide between these two alternative explanations but it is important to be clear that at least two explanations are possible.

An early experiment (Dement, 1960) did indicate that deprivation of AS might lead to psychotic episodes, but subsequent research has failed to reproduce this finding. Moreover, certain antidepressant drugs in common use in psychiatry have the ability to eliminate AS completely for many months without any obvious ill effect on the patient. It seems, therefore, that lack of AS is not, in itself, harmful. In addition, a few studies of total sleep deprivation have reported occasional hallucinations in their subjects. Most studies do not observe them and it must not be assumed that hallucinations are an automatic consequence of sleep deprivation. Murray (1965, chs 6 and 7), who gives a very full account of the psychological effects of total sleep deprivation, attempts to explain its effect in terms of motivational changes experienced by sleep-deprived people. The conflict experienced during the vigil generates frustration which results in irritability and anxiety. When the sleep-deprived individual reaches the point where he is dipping frequently into partial sleep, then the psychotic phenomena appear. These phenomena can be encouraged by the social situation and the expectations of the staff running the experiment. Murray quotes evidence that psychotic phenomena can be observed as a result of starvation, thirst, salt depletion, oxygen deficiency and sensory deprivation and suggests that the psychotic phenomena are the result of a severe frustration of a common motivational mechanism and are not necessarily directly caused by a physiological deficit resulting from lack of sleep.

Function of sleep

Before we were aware of much of the detailed information given above, the job of assigning a function to sleep seemed straightforward. The most popular candidate was the role of recuperation from physical or mental fatigue, and an approachable summary of the arguments in favour at that time is given in Murray (1965, ch. 2). While the exact function was never pinpointed with any certainty, there appeared to be little reason to dissent from this general view. More recently the realization that sleep involves at least two (and possibly more) major types of state has led to a new generation of theories which assign a different recuperative function to each state. Because of the profusion of functions which have been proposed we can do no more than summarize the most important theories here.

AS has received most theoretical attention, probably because of its intriguing nature and its relative novelty. There is a broad split of theories into two main camps, psychological and biological. The psychological group of functions were most popular when it was believed that AS deprivation led to madness since AS was assigned the role of syphoning off excess drive and acting as an unconscious pressure release valve following the Freudian view. Such theories have become less fashionable recently, but they retain an acceptable presence in the form of memory consolidation views. These rely on evidence that some types of material, memorized before going to sleep, are better recalled on arousal if AS is present during the interval before waking. In a similar vein, it is believed, by some, that AS permits the reworking of old memories and unsolved problems. These theories are sympathetically reviewed by Cartwright (1977) who also bases her argument on the small amount of AS found in schizophrenics and the flat, eventless nature of their reported dreams.

Biological theories of AS function subdivide into two broad types, emphasizing either neural stimulation or repair functions. Stimulation theories point to the activated nature of AS and suggest that a repeated shake-up during sleep must be a good antidote to the lethargy of QS. This could involve exercise of the nervous system generally (Ephron and Carrington, 1966) or the delicate muscles which control the eyes (Berger, 1969). We have already discussed the suggestion (Roffwarg et al., 1966) that AS may serve to stimulate the growth of brain cells in the foetus. Snyder (1966) believed AS stimulated the brain into a stage of preparedness so as to benefit maximally from the brief arousals which typically follow AS episodes. Major repair function theories (Hartmann, 1973; Oswald, 1974), on the other hand, have concentrated on protein metabolism which appears to be increased at this time and would certainly be useful in the growing foetus too.

By comparison QS has received little attention from the theorists, possibly as the result of a tacit assumption that QS had inherited many of the recuperation functions previously assigned to sleep in general. Both Hartmann (1973) and Oswald (1974) argue in favour of growth or repair of general body tissues at this time, although Hartmann believes that important biochemical operations also take place in brain cells in preparation for the protein metabolism which will take place later during AS. Oswald draws attention to the extra secretion of growth hormone during DQS soon after sleep onset as well as to the increase in amounts of DQS he observed during periods of total food starvation. It is important to note that theories of the function of QS usually refer only to DQS which occupies up to 80 per cent of the sleep of the laboratory rat but usually less than 25 per cent of the sleep of adult man. LQS which occupies approximately half of man's sleeping time is rarely mentioned even though, for this reason alone, we might argue that it is a very important type of sleep. It is hoped that future theories of the recuperative function of sleep will be more complete in their coverage, since it is unlikely that man requires so much less recovery than the rat, if indeed recovery is the main function of sleep.

When considering the status of existing theories of function, we need to be aware of ambiguities in the meanings of the words 'function' and 'need'. For example, my feet may become hardened by regular walking. Can we therefore say that the function of walking is to harden the feet? Normally, the function of walking is to get to places, although we might also benefit later from toughened feet. In this sense, the significance of increased protein metabolism during AS or a

122 Brain, Behaviour and Evolution

reduction in the deterioration of recent memories is also ambiguous. Are they incidental but useful consequences of the sleep state, or do they point to the prime function which originally dictated the necessity for such a sleep state and determined the fine details of its operation? The question is not easy to resolve on existing evidence.

Similarly, the expression 'need for sleep' has ambiguities. We all possess a neurological mechanism which regulates our sleeping and waking times. It introduces drowsiness and an increased desire for sleep which itensifies and persists until we have finally yielded by allowing sleep to take over. The operation of this mechanism induces in us a felt 'need for sleep' which is psychological in nature. It also produces a practical 'need for sleep' in the sense that the drowsiness will not permit us to work effectively towards our other goals until we have permitted sleep to take place. However, there is also a third meaning which centres on the need for the mechanism itself which switches us on and off and meddles with our psychological states.

An animal approaching hibernation neatly illustrates these different meanings. When discussing the function of hibernation, we are concerned solely with the need for the control system; almost certainly this is not for the purposes of recuperation, but it is a behavioural and physiological strategem intended to avoid the rigours of winter. When talking about sleep, we tend to get our meanings of 'need' mixed up. We often argue that late-night feelings of fatigue are evidence that our batteries have run down when really it only signifies that the sleep control mechanism is beginning to apply pressure to get us to go to bed. We also argue that because we cannot usefully do anything until after we have had a sleep, then we must need sleep to 'recover' from the ill effects of wakefulness. Of course, this does not logically follow and a better analogy might be sportsmen waiting for a shower to pass before continuing with the game.

We cannot infer that sleep promotes recovery simply because we feel tired in the evening. It is the sleep control mechanism which makes us feel tired. The question we must ask is whether the period of immobility called sleep is essential for recovery of some particular deficit which has accumulated during wakefulness. To answer this question we need to specify the deficit and then provide evidence that sleep is the only means of correcting it. In my view such evidence has not been forthcoming and the general faith in recuperation theories is largely dependent on fairly circumstantial grounds such as the effects of sleep deprivation. But this, as we have already seen, has a respectable alternative explanation which does not involve physiological recuperation.

This does not mean that sleep may have no function. On the contrary, students of animal behaviour have always understood that sleep control mechanisms help to schedule periods of activity and inactivity to suit circadian changes in environmental pressures and opportunities. In this sense, sleep and hibernation have much in common. It is certainly clear from Figure 5.1 that most animals do not need a full twenty-four hours to carry out essential business, although species vary in the amount of spare time they have available. Sleep serves to keep an animal quiet, inconspicuous and out of harm's way during this spare time, thus minimizing predation and producing a saving of energy expenditure compared with non-stop physical activity.

The function is also recognized by sleep theorists and the benefits are clearly understood (Murray, 1965; Webb, 1975; Meddis, 1977). What is at issue is whether this function is alone sufficient to explain the existence of the sleep control mechanism, as I believe, or whether it is necessary to add further reasons in the form of recovery processes. The issue is important because it affects fundamentally our view of what sleep really is; a time of immobile retreat from the rigours of the environment or a time of physiological and psychological recovery. Whatever we decide will profoundly influence the kind of attitudes we have to our own sleep, the kind of research we carry out and the kind of treatments we create for sleep disorders such as insomnia.

It will also influence a decision on whether sleep is really necessary. Figure 5.1 indicates that there are many animal species which seem to get by with very much less sleep than man. How can they get by with less if the purpose of sleep is recovery? Not all people sleep for seven hours a day. Some sleep for very much less and a few people called 'nonsomniacs' hardly sleep at all whilst remaining perfectly fit. As part of my research I have sought out these very short sleepers either personally or by sifting reports (Meddis, 1977) and it is now clear that some individuals do get by happily and healthily on an average of one hour or less of sleep per night.

One lady claimed to sleep for an average of fifty minutes per night. When we studied her in the laboratory for five days with round-the-clock surveillance and EEG monitoring of her sleep, she averaged sixty-seven minutes per night which is near enough to her original claim. Such individuals are difficult to understand from the point of view of a recuperative theory of sleep, but they agree quite well with the notion that the sleep control mechanism merely serves to schedule activity and promote periods of immobility where appropriate. In the case of the short sleepers, the mechanism does not function normally but the consequent reduction in their sleeping time. does them no harm.

Conclusion

In a single chapter it is difficult to give an unbiased account of everything which is happening in a rapidly changing field. Our biases and theories determine which data we find important and which can be safely omitted. Another author would certainly have painted a different picture. Fortunately there are now a number of readable books which cover the same ground from different angles but in much greater detail, for example Cartwright (1977), Hartmann (1973), Oswald (1974) and Webb (1975).

All authors would nevertheless agree that our image of sleep has changed dramatically in the last few years and is still changing. Sleep is now much more complex and is more deeply rooted in biology than ever before. It seems likely that a better understanding of its biological nature will provide the key to understanding experiential, behavioural and electrophysiological aspects which, hitherto, have been dealt with separately. For example, an acceptable theory of the evolution of AS should provide a good basis for better explanations of the origins of dreams and a detailed understanding of the working of the 'sleep instinct' could explain many phenomena such as drowsiness and raised response thresholds during sleep. However, we may only be allowed to reap this harvest if we are prepared to abandon some old and time-honoured notions of the nature and function of sleep in favour of newer and less familiar perspectives.

References

Adams, K. and Oswald, I. (1977) Sleep is for tissue restoration. *Journal of the Royal College of Physicians* 11: 376–88.

Allison, T. (1970) The evolution of sleep. *Natural History* 79: 56–65.

Allison, T. and Cicchetti, D. V. (1976) Sleep in mammals: ecological and constitutional correlates. *Science 194*: 732–4.

Berger, R. (1969) Oculomotor control: a possible function for REM sleep. *Psychological Review 76*: 144–64.

Cartwright, R. D. (1977) *Night Life*. Englewood Cliffs, N. J.: Prentice-Hall

Dement, W. C. (1960) The effect of dream deprivation. *Science 131*: 1705–7.

Dement, W. C. (1972) *Some Must Watch While Some Must Sleep*. San Francisco: Freeman.

Ephron, H. S. and Carrington, P. (1966). Rapid eye movement sleep and cortical homeostasis. *Psychological Review 73*: 500–26.

Freud, S. (1955) *The Interpretation of Dreams*. New York: Basic Books.

Hartmann, E. L. (1973) *The Functions of Sleep*. New Haven: Yale University Press.

Horne, J. A. (in press) Human sleep and body restitution. *Experientia*.

Meddis, R. (1975) On the function of sleep. *Animal Behaviour 23*: 676–91.

Meddis, R. (1977) *The Sleep Instinct*. London: Routledge and Kegan Paul.

Murray, E. J. (1965) *Sleep Dreams and Arousal*. New York: Appleton-Century-Crofts.

Oswald, I. (1974) *Sleep*. Harmondsworth: Penguin.

Rechtschaffen, A. and Kales, A. (eds) (1968) *A Manual of Standardized Terminology, Techniques and Scoring System for Sleep Stages of Human Subjects*. Washington D.C.: US Government Printing Office.

Robinson, T. E., Kramis, R. C. and Vanderwolf, C. H. (1977) Two types of cerebral activation during active sleep: relations to behaviour. *Brain Research 124*: 544–9.

Roffwarg, H., Muzio, J. and Dement, W. (1966) Ontogenetic development of human sleep-dream cycle. *Science 152*: 604–18.

Snyder, F. (1966) Toward an evolutionary theory of dreaming. *American Journal of Psychiatry 123*: 121–36.

Tinbergen, N. (1951) *The Study of Instinct*. London: Oxford University Press.

Webb, W. B. (1975) *Sleep, The Gentle Tyrant*. Englewood Cliffs, N.J.: Prentice-Hall.

6   Brain size and intelligence: a comparative perspective

I. Steele Russell

Introduction

In any consideration of comparative neural mechanisms of behaviour the general characteristics of the brain reveal a common pattern throughout the vertebrate series. Beginning with early fish and moving through reptiles, the brains of birds and mammals follow somewhat different paths from this common origin (see Introduction and Chapter 2 of this volume). In very general terms, during vertebrate evolution there is a progressive increase in the size and complexity of the brain relative to the spinal cord. At the same time there is a relatively greater increase in the development of the cerebrum. In mammals this trend is further continued by an increase in the size of the cerebral cortex in comparison with the rest of the brain. It is traditionally believed that this reflects two general tendencies. First, that the increase in brain size is related to intelligence in the form of the increasing complexity and adaptiveness of behaviour. Second, there is the notion of encephalization or corticalization of function, which is the belief that as the brain evolves from early fishes to modern mammals such as man, functions that were originally controlled by lower brain structures are taken over by the cerebrum and the cortex (see Chapters 2 and 7 of this volume).

Anatomically one of the most obvious signs of encephalization in mammals is the increase in the amount of neocortex. Insectivore brains are relatively small and have little cortex; they are more or less lissencephalic (smooth-brained) having few neocortical folds. With the evolution of relatively larger brains and more neocortex, there is an obvious development in the extensiveness of the folds of the cortex. Both the depth and frequency of the convolutions increase in all mammals as the size and complexity of their brain increases. Whilst the causes and mechanisms of cortical folding are not clear, it does permit a greater increase in surface area without a large increase in volume (Leboucq, 1929). None the less comparisons of the brain of prosimians, old and new world monkeys, apes and man reveal that the extent of convolution of the brain increases not only as a phylogenetic trend but is also highly correlated with brain size (Radinsky, 1975).

It is important when considering these evolutionary changes involved in encephalization, that one does not create the impression that they are solely restricted to the brain. Major changes also occur in the organization of the spinal cord. The intrinsic mechanisms that determine temporal and spatial patterning of neural 'commands' to the muscles are the major component of spinal function. These mechanisms are relatively autonomous in lower vertibrates. Although there can be limited autonomy of visceral reflexes in higher vertibrates, none the less cephalic dominance over spinal cord function is a major evolutionary trend. This can be seen in a variety of ways. Higher vertibrates show less normal autonomy of the cord and have a greater dependency on the brain in the control of spinal reflexes in locomotion. This is related morphologically in the progressive increase in the proportion of white matter (fibres) in the spinal cord of these animals. Further the effect of transsection of the cord in higher mammals is to produce a state of 'spinal shock' below the section, where the animal is both inactive and profoundly non-responsive. This condition dissipates within days or weeks in man, hours in the cat, and is not reliably discernible in amphibians or fish. A further change that also occurs in the evolution of the brain is the development of the automatic nervous system, which plays such a considerable role in the homeostatic mechanisms of homeothermy. Although there is some innervation of the viscera in the lowest vertebrates, it increases enormously in extent and complexity in higher vertibrates such as birds and mammals. A well-defined sympathetic nervous system is found in fish but there is no double innervation of the viscera by opposed sympathetic and para-sympathetic action. This dual control system first emerges in amphibians and reptiles. In warm blooded animals such as birds and mammals this system increases in complexity and comes under the central control of the hypothalamus.

The present chapter examines the empirical basis for the principle of encephalization and considers in detail the evidence for the evolutionary emergence of enlarged brains in excess of the requirements of body size. It also considers the related issues of whether or not the increase in brain size is due in the main to the increase in proportionate size of the neocortex. Finally, the relationship between brain size or brain development and intelligence is examined.

Brain size and intelligence in man

Such considerations as these have led to the belief that there is a relationship between the size of the human brain and amount of intelligence. This question has been approached by considering extreme cases, where the brains of eminent men are compared to those of mental defectives. Many men of outstanding ability have indeed been the possessors in life of large brains. Kant's brain is reputed to have weighed 1600 gms and Schiller's brain was 1785 gms. Cuvier's brain was larger still, having a weight of 1830 gms. The largest human brain that was reliably measured was that of Turgenev with a weight of 2012 gms. These are to be compared to the average weight of 1440 gms for the male human brain (Blinkov and Glazer, 1968). On the other hand many eminent men seem to have possessed either decidedly average-sized brains or brains that were markedly underdeveloped in size. For example Gauss's brain weighed 1492 gms and Liebig's brain was 1352 gms. Both Gambetta and Hausmann had below average brains at 1246 gms and 1226 gms respectively – this does not appear to have had any adverse effect on their careers! Most striking is the example of Anatole France who was found to possess a brain weighing only 1017 grams, which is a weight usually associated with idiocy!

These selected examples illustrate dramatically the general point that within a single species there is no simple relationship between brain size and intelligence or intellectual achievement. They also show the dangers of such arbitrary selectivity in correlating brain and behaviour. The weight of the brain can be affected by many artifacts of measurement as well as by such variables as age, sex and stature. For example, congestion of the blood vessels and the inclusion of the cerebral membranes of the dura and pia mater can increase the weight by 60 to 100 gms. The presence of degenerative changes and atrophy could cause a marked reduction in cerebral weight.

At birth the human brain weighs approximately 380 gms and is 12·3 per cent of body weight (Muhlman, 1957). By two years of age the brain is 1024 gms and thereafter the rate of growth is less dramatic up to the seventh year when the brain weighs 1350 gms. There is a very gradual increase in size until the age of twenty when the the brain reaches its average maximum size of 1444 gms for men and 1228 gms for women. As the average body structure and weight of the female are smaller than the male, when the brain is compared as a proportion of the body weight then the two sexes are equal with 2.43 per cent for men and 2·41 per cent for women. For both sexes from the age of thirty onwards there is a continuous diminution in brain weight until, by the age of eighty, the average is 1280 gms and 1116 gms for men and women respectively. After the age of thirty there is an annual loss of 2–3 gms in brain weight for both sexes. The rate is not constant, however, as it accelerates after the age of sixty.

Considering the brain weights of outstanding individuals in isolation is a highly arbitrary and not a meaningful practice. In general most individuals do not achieve intellectual eminence or recognition unless they live to a fairly advanced age. Thus there is a selection factor operating to underestimate the true size of their brain due to the effects of aging. For example, in the case of Anatole France who died at the age of eighty, if corrections are made for aging ($50 \times 3·28$) and the weight of brain membranes (60 gms), then his brain weight at maturity was probably 1240 gms. This is not discrepant as it falls within two standard deviations of the mean (SD = 110 gms for men). Furthermore, when the average brain weight was calculated for mental defectives, it was not found to differ significantly from the normal although the variance was larger (Penrose, 1949). Similarly, comparisons of the average head size of groups of people of superior, average and below average ability reveal that statistically there is no significant correlation between intelligence and head size.

Comparative studies of the evolution of the brain

Considering the changes in size and complexity of the brain over the entire vertebrate series, it is obvious that some relationship between

Table 6.1   Brain weights in gms of 21 mammals arranged in descending order

1	Whale	6800	8	Ox	493	15	Cat	25
2	Elephant	4717	9	Chimp	440	16	Squirrel monkey	25
3	Dolphin	1735	10	Wild pig	178	17	Rabbit	10
4	Man	1444	11	Sheep	140	18	Squirrel	6
5	Walrus	1126	12	Macaque	106	19	Marmoset	7
6	Camel	762	13	Dog	79	20	Rat	2·36
7	Horse	532	14	Fox	53	21	Mouse	0·43

brain size and intelligence exists. Differences in size of body are not, however, without effect on the size of the brain. For example, in comparing animals of different species either within the same order or not, some allowance has to be made for body size before looking for a relationship between brain size and intelligence.

This point is made dramatically when we consider a table of mammalian brain weights where there is an obvious disproportionate bias due to the size of the animal (see Table 6.1). Like other organs

Table 6.2   Ratio of brain weight to body weight of 21 mammals arranged in ascending order

1	Squirrel monkey	1:26	8	Fox	1:87	15	Sheep	1:394
2	Marmoset	1:29	9	Cat	1:120	16	Camel	1:525
3	Mouse	1:38	10	Chimpanzee	1:128	17	Walrus	1:592
4	Man	1:44	11	Rat	1:152	18	Elephant	1:645
5	Squirrel	1:53	12	Dog	1:170	19	Horse	1:692
6	Dolphin	1:82	13	Rabbit	1:300	20	Whale	1:854
7	Macaque	1:82	14	Wild pig	1:314	21	Ox	1:1339

the brain is large or small in different species according to whether the body is large or small. Large animal species tend to have large livers, hearts, kidneys and lungs as well as large brains. It is necessary to correct for this body size factor to see whether or not there are any residual differences in relative brain development of different species. Merely correcting the brain weights by dividing them by body weights, however, does not solve the problem since the ratio itself decreases with the increase in body weight. When species are ordered according to their proportionate size of brain to body weight, there is a tendency to produce an overcompensation for the body size factor (see Table 6.2). Thus, for the squirrel monkey the brain constitutes 1/26th of the whole body weight whereas for the ox it is only one part in 1,339 of the total weight. There is a significant inverse correlation with body weight which radically favours the smaller animals and totally overshadows any relationship between brain size and intelligence. Man is ranked below the mouse and above the squirrel, and the chimpanzee is placed well below the macaque and only marginally superior to the rat.

An early attempt to resolve this difficulty was made by Snell (1891) who observed that the size of the brain was related not to the weight (or volume) of the body but to its surface area. He argued that the surface of the body would be the more appropriate measure to take for the correction because of the importance of body surface area for general metabolism. Dubois (1897) developed the first index of encephalization based on Snell's suggestion that there is a significant relationship between brain size (E) and body surface area (A). As the surface area is related by a power function to the body weight (P), this enabled Snell to express the relationship between brain size and body surface area by the allometric equation $E = kP^a$, where the exponent a is a constant (phylogenetic constant) and k varies across species and is the cephalization coefficient. Dubois suggested that the true rationale for the relationship between the brain and the body surface is that the surface of the skin is the site of sense organs and is therefore richly supplied with sensory nerves. As the function of the brain is to regulate the body in relation to the outside world, there should be some discernible relation between the amount of skin surface area and brain size.

Comparing animals of equal 'cephalic development' such as a domestic cat and a lion Dubois was to derive an *ad hoc* method of determining the value of a. For example, a cat has a length of about 60 cms whereas a lion would be 200 cms. The linear measure (L) of the lion is thus about 3·3 times that of the cat. Furthermore its surface area (A) is about 11 times that of a cat and its volume (V) is about 36 times that of a cat. The lion's brain weighs approximately 240 gms. If there was a direct relationship between brain weight (E) and body weight (P) (represented by body volume V), then 240 gms divided by 36 would give an estimated brain size of 7 gms for a lion of a body size similar to that of a cat. If, however, we divide the lion's brain weight by 11, thus correcting not by volume but by surface area, we obtain an estimated brain size of 22 gms which is much closer to the real size of a cat's brain at 25 gms.

Snell (1891) had argued that in pairs of animals of similar form it is possible to assume that body surface areas (A and A′) will be in the same proportion as the squares of the linear measures (L² and L′²). In dealing with body surfaces of differing species, however, it is much more convenient to utilize body weights to represent body volumes (V and V′). It should be recalled that body weight (P) is identical to body volume (V) when a specific gravity of 1·0 is assumed for body tissues. The linear measure can be estimated from the cube root of the volumes. The surface areas can then be obtained from the square of such values, hence $a = \frac{2}{3}$. Thus the comparison of brain weights to body surface could be obtained by:

$$\frac{E}{A} = \frac{E'}{A'} = \frac{E}{L^2} = \frac{E'}{L'^2} = \frac{E}{V^{2/3}} = \frac{E'}{V'^{2/3}}$$

The last equality is the most convenient as it entails components that are easily and accurately measured (i.e. as brain weight for E and body weight for V).

Dubois with his method of paired comparisons undertook to determine empirically the value of the exponent a, which had been rationally determined by Snell. Thus: $\frac{E}{V}a = \frac{E'}{V'}a$ is equivalent to $\frac{E}{E'} = \frac{V}{V'}$ a. Transforming this logarithmically and solving for a, we see that $a = \frac{\log E - \log E'}{\log V - \log V'}$. Using this expression Dubois calculated values for *suitably* related pairs of animals such as the lion and the domestic cat. The cat has a brain weight of 25 gms and body weight of 3000 gms, which compares to a brain weight of 240 gms and 15,000 gms body weight for the lion. Using these values in the above equation it is found that $a = 0.5782$, which is less than that expected on *a priori* grounds by Snell. Taking other suitable pairs of animals that are both related and differ greatly in size, Dubois was able to calculate an entire series of a values. In all cases the value was found to be less than 0·666 and had an average of 0.5613 ± 0.0176.

As a appeared to have the same approximate value for all mammals, Dubois generalized his original statement. Thus from $\frac{E}{V^a} = \frac{E'}{V'^a}$ it became $E/V^a = k$, and $E'/V'^a = k$, or $E = kV^a$ and $E' = kV'^a$ where k is a constant which is the same for the pair of animals considered. As a has the same value for all mammals and if the weight of the body and the brain are known for any mammal, then k will have a value which will vary across species reflecting the degree of development or complexity of the brain. The parameter k for this reason was called the cephalization coefficient, and is given by: $k = E/V^a$.

A selection of k values calculated for a variety of mammals is shown in Table 6.3. The ranking which emerges on the basis of these values is clearly more in line with the ranking which we might intuitively make on the basis of assumed intelligence. None the less when some of the details are considered, certain positions appear unusual, as for example the low placing of the marmoset, which is a New World primate.

Table 6.3   Estimated k values in 21 mammals arranged in descending order

1	Man	2.8419	8	Walrus	0·6060	15	Sheep	0·3057
2	Dolphin	2·2212	9	Camel	0·5464	16	Cat	0·2794
3	Whale	1·0863	10	Fox	0·4646	17	Ox	0·2669
4	Elephant	1·0819	11	Horse	0·3998	18	Squirrel	0·2343
5	Chimpanzee	0·9482	12	Wild pig	0·3848	19	Rabbit	0·1118
6	Squirrel monkey	0·6709	13	Dog	0·3811	20	Rat	0·896
7	Macaque	0·6509	14	Marmoset	0·3577	21	Mouse	0·0826

Considering that Dubois had constructed his cephalization index by assuming that animals of related species had an identical degree of encephalization, it is not surprising that the ordering was arbitrary due to the *ad hoc* nature of the method of evaluation of a. Indeed the selection of related animals as 'suitable' pairs is crucial. Entirely different values are obtained when a tiger and lion are paired $(a = ·4421)$ or a puma and serval $(a = ·6672)$. Von Bonin (1937) attempted to resolve this situation by adopting a more legitimate statistical approach to the problem. He undertook the orthodox approach of curve fitting a straight line to the logarithms of the brain and body weight of over 100 mammals. Using a regression analysis, he was able to estimate a at approximately $2/3$, which was in agreement with Snell's rational value. Later work by Scholl (1948) showed, however, that a was not a demonstrable constant for related species of animals. He found that the phylogenetic constant for four species of macaque monkeys was low where $a = 0·18$. Furthermore, Scholl also demonstrated that when individuals within a species were compared, extremely low estimates of a were obtained. This work discredited the notion of deriving indices of cephalic development. The calculation of cephalic indices for individuals of a species is both questionable and incompatible with the conceptual rationale of an index of cephalization. It is clear that such an index would only legitimately and reliably discriminate across very broad groups of animals. Where a wide range of species is compared then the differences *between* species are consistently greater than the variation *within* species. Hence an index of encephalization could have both reliability and validity as an indicator of comparative brain development. Where there is a considerable degree of overlap in species, however, as in Scholl's study of four species of macaque monkeys, then the differences *within* species will be as great as those *between* species. When this is the case, there is no possibility of discerning reliable or valid species differences on logical grounds.

In order to minimize this error it is essential to survey a representative sample of vertebrate brain-body weights. Previous efforts have been flawed by the use of arbitrary material selected from different sources containing several artifacts, such as failing to distinguish between specimens that were juvenile rather than adult, to distinguish the emaciated from the healthy, or to identify errors due to collection and preservation procedures. There are advantages in being able to draw on material collected by a single team of investigators whose methods are therefore reasonably constant across species. The most comprehensive approximation to this is the material provided by Crile and Quiring (1940) who reported the living weights of 3581 vertebrate specimens. Using this material Jerison (1973) has compiled brain-body data for 198 different vertebrate species (see Figure 6.1) consisting of 94 mammalian (including 18 primate species), 52 avian, 20 reptile and 32 fish species.

Unfortunately even with such a broad phylogenetic spectrum is was not possible to report values for each species in terms of a representative mean and standard deviation. Accordingly Jerison arbitrarily selected individual values of species from the Crile and Quiring material which agreed with the range of values given in standard zoological texts. Furthermore, wherever possible the weights for the heaviest specimen were used. The rationale for this was that the heavier animal was more representative of the phenotype when dealing with material taken from the wild by hunting and fishing. There is under these circumstances a collection bias favouring the sampling

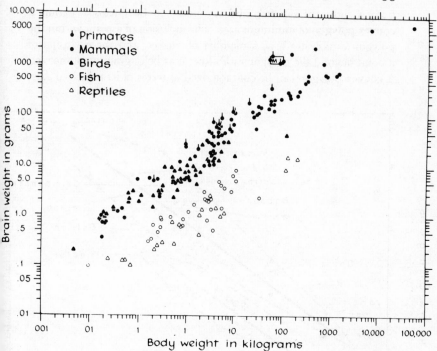

Fig. 6.1   Brain – body weights of 198 vertebrate species collected by Crile and Quiring (1940), graphed on log-coordinates. From Jerison 1973.

of the younger or weaker animals as they are more likely to be caught.

From Figure 6.1 it is apparent that living vertebrates readily separate into two broad groups with respect to brain development. There are what Jerison refers to as the 'lower' vertebrates including fish and reptiles, and the 'higher' vertebrate group of avians and mammals (see Introduction and Chapter 2 of this volume). Each species is represented by a single point, with the exception of man which is represented by the rectangle M. This contains the extreme values of the Crile and Quiring sample of 42 male human-body weights. The brains ranged from the lightest of 1130 gms to the heaviest of 1570 gms with body weights ranging from 36,000 gms to 95,000 gms.

Jerison has analysed these data using the method of minimum convex polygons which enables a set of points – the brain-body weights of say fish and reptiles – to be enclosed within a convex polygon of minimum area. The inclusion of a point within the polygon establishes it as a member of the set, and the exclusion of a point beyond the polygon establishes it as belonging to another set. A convex polygon can be characterized in terms of its principal axis,

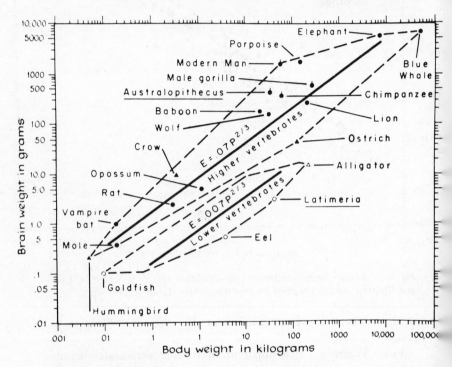

Fig. 6.2   Selected data points from Figure 1. Minimum convex polygons are shown by dashed lines, enclosing visually placed central axes with slopes of 0·666. From Jerison 1973.

which is equivalent to placing a regression line. Jerison argues that this method enables a map to be drawn for the level of brain development of species within any class of animals such as mammals. Figure 6.2 illustrates the use of this analysis on the data given in Figure 6.1, where it can be seen that there are two distinct non-overlapping polygons. The polygon for 'higher' vertebrates in fact contains a natural grouping of mammals and avians. When these two classes were separately analysed they were found to have almost completely overlapping polygons. The fish and reptiles similarly formed the second grouping of 'lower' vertebrates. The straight lines within each polygon in Figure 6.2 represent the principal axis which is used to represent the regions of the polygon. The allometric equation $E = kP^a$ is used to provide a line of best-fit. The value of the parameter a was arbitrarily selected by Jerison to have the value of $2/3$ or $0 \cdot 666$ in order to retain the surface area:volume relationship of Snell. This has the further advantage, therefore, that all principal axes will have parallel slopes, which gives the impression (Figure 6.2) that the increase in relative brain size between 'lower' and 'higher' vertebrates was of a tenfold order. The extent of the vertical displacement is given by the intercept parameter k which has a value of $0 \cdot 007$ for 'lower' vertebrates and $0 \cdot 07$ for 'higher' vertebrates. It is important to note that Jerison *did not* use any mathematical curve fitting procedure such as the method of least squares to place his principle axes. They were chosen to have equal slopes (that is $a = 0 \cdot 666$) and were then visually placed through 'the approximate centroid of each array of data' (Jerison, 1973, p. 49). However the earlier analyses of Quiring (1941), who used traditional regression techniques on the same data, produced essentially the same conclusions with regard to both the separation of species into two main groups of 'lower' and 'higher' vertebrates and the tenfold increase in relative brain size of the 'higher' over the 'lower' vertebrates. Despite this the *objective estimates* of the phyletic constant vary considerably. Quiring (1941) obtained a value of $0 \cdot 541$ for all vertebrates; Jerison reports values of $0 \cdot 69$ for mammals, $0 \cdot 56$ for avians, $0 \cdot 50$ for fish and $0 \cdot 62$ for reptiles.

Using the equation $E = kP^a$ it is possible to calculate an expected brain size (E_e) for any given species where $E = E_e$ is assumed. The value of the intercept parameter k varies according to the class of vertebrate concerned; for fish and reptiles $k = 0 \cdot 007$, for avians it is equal to $0 \cdot 07$ and for mammals it is $0 \cdot 12$. Jerison uses this estimate of expected brain size to provide a measure of what he calls the *encephalization quotient* (EQ). This is obtained by expressing the real or true brain size (E_t) of a species as a proportion of the expected brain size for an animal of equivalent body size. Thus the equation $EQ = E_t/E_e$ or $EQ = E_t/kP^a$ would estimate the quotient of any species where the brain and body size are known. Thus in the case of the previous example of a domestic cat, with an average body weight of 3000 gms and a brain size of 25 gms, the expected brain size would be: $E_e = 0.12 \ (3000)^{2/3} = 24.95$. Therefore the $EQ = E_t/E_e$ $= 25/24.95 = 1.0$.

Arranging our series of animals in order according to their EQ value shows that certain significant changes have occurred (see Table 6.4). It can be seen that the various primates have been concentrated together, displacing the elephant and the whale; and the

Table 6.4 Encephalization Quotients (EQs) of 21 mammals arranged in descending order

1 Man	7·4416	8 Marmoset	1·7063	15 Cat	1·0021
2 Dolphin	5·3055	9 Fox	1·5920	16 Horse	0·8640
3 Chimp	2·4865	10 Walrus	1·2303	17 Sheep	0·8075
4 Squirrel					
monkey	2·3228	11 Camel	1·1707	18 Ox	0·5424
5 Macaque	2·0865	12 Dog	1·1677	19 Mouse	0·5033
6 Elephant	1·8717	13 Squirrel	1·1033	20 Rat	0·4029
7 Whale	1·7560	14 Wild pig	1·0141	21 Rabbit	0·4008

squirrel has been favoured by a dramatic increase in relative position. As to whether this ordering has significance in terms of relative increase in intelligence or degree of encephalization is questionable. The ordering in terms of EQ values may *intuitively* match the relative level of evolution of the brain for the various mammalian species. Certainly it should reflect the most rational way of expressing the extent to which the brain has developed over and above the body size requirements. The fact that primates as a group in our list of mammals appear to be amongst the most highly encephalized mammals is in agreement with the fact that some of them are also amongst the least specialized and the most adaptive of mammals with a highly generalized anatomy. Not only their learning and reasoning ability but also their adaptability to a wide range of climates, terrain and foods reflect this.

Change in the size of the brain with evolution is only one aspect of the situation. There are also other factors such as changes in cerebral organization with increasing size, changes in the types of cell with encephalization, and changes in the complexity of neural networks. The question is to what extent does increasing encephalization entail both quantitative and qualitative changes. From many points of view, there has been a tendency to regard it as mainly a quantitative change. Considering 'higher' vertebrates (birds and mammals) as a whole, it is true that the same fundamental ground plan of the brain applies to both major classes. However the tendency to regard the avian brain as a simpler version of the mammalian brain is both erroneous and misleading. The fact that the neocortex has evolved in mammalian and marsupial brains and not in avian ones is only part of the difference between them. At the same time there has been the development of the Wulst or hyper-striatum in avians which has no counterpart in the mammalian brain (see Chapter 2).Thus claims by some comparative psychologists that an avian brain can be heuristically considered as a 'natural' decorticate or limbic preparation are mistaken. Indeed it is debatable whether changes in the encephalization within say the mammalian order are profitably considered as uniform quantitative variations on the same theme. For example, there is no Wulst in cat as there is in pigeon; hence it is possible that in vision certain functions are handled differently in various species and thereby organized differently. Pattern and distance vision need not have the same method of data processing and so could be handled by different structures across species. It is likely that pattern vision is processed differently in rats, cats and monkeys and this fact produces different data proces-sing requirements of the brain.

Within the mammalian order the most obvious change in brain development is the progressive increase in cortex from lissencephalic (smooth) brains to convoluted brains. A note of caution should be made, however, with regard to the notion that the transition from smooth to convoluted cortex separates 'lower' mammals from 'higher' ones. Many primates, particularly the small primates, are lissen-cephalic; also the echidna, a monotreme (see Introduction to this volume), has a highly convoluted brain.

The amount of cortex as a proportion of the brain increases pro-gressively throughout mammalian series. Harman (1957) estimates that the proportion was 30 per cent in rodents, 43 per cent in carnivores and 52 per cent in primates. More dramatic is the propor-tionate increase of neocortex compared to archicortex, paleocortex and intermediate cortex (see Chapter 2 of this volume). The lowest proportion is in insectivores such as the hedgehog with 52 per cent of neocortex; the rabbit has 56 per cent, the rat 62 per cent, the dog 84 per cent, marmoset 85 per cent, macaque 93 per cent, chimpanzee 93 per cent, man 96 per cent and dolphin 98 per cent.

The relationship between the amount of cortex and the size of the brain has been extensively investigated over a large series of mammals.

Harman (1957) found a close relationship between cortical volume and brain volume for a mammalian series ranging through rodents, ungulates, carnivores and primates. A similar relationship between brain volume and cortical surface area for a broad mammal spectrum was found by Elias and Schwartz (1969). This relationship is perhaps most convincingly demonstrated when examined over a related series of mammals by Stephan et al. (1970). The progressive increase in cortex is traced from the living 'ancestral' forms of insectivores through prosimians, monkeys and apes to man (Figure 6.3). Not only does the amount of cortex increase throughout the series, but it does so as an orderly function of brain mass. In prosimians the cortex is 50 per cent of brain mass, in monkeys 68

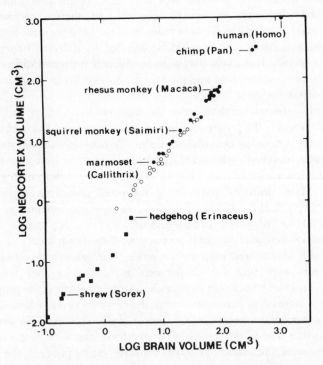

Fig. 6.3 Relationship between volume of neocortex and brain size in 10 basal insectivores (squares), 18 prosimians (open circles) and 21 anthropoids (solid circles). Note that the primates have more cortex for their brain size than insectivores. From Radinsky 1975.

per cent, in apes 74 per cent and in man 80 per cent.

Although man has proportionately more cortex than other primates, it is important to note that there is no discontinuity in the series and that he has only the amount of cortex that is expected for a primate of his brain size. Finally, what is also impressive about these findings is that the amount of cortex is exactly determined by the size of the brain and does not have to be expressed as a function of the degree of complexity of brain convolutions.

A second striking change in the mammalian brain is the evolutionary changes in the balance of the sensory systems. There is a progressive decrease in the use of olfaction and an increase in the importance of vision. This is particularly true of primates (Stephan, 1969; Radinsky, 1975). Not only does the olfactory bulb decrease in prosimians compared with insectivores, with most species having 90 per cent of the size of the olfactory bulb that would be expected of a basal insectivore of equivalent body weight; there is a further decrease in the relative size of olfactory bulbs of simians to approximately 20 per cent to 10 per cent of that of the insectivore. Finally, with the anthropoid apes and man, there is a further reduction to less than 5 per cent. This fall from grace in the importance of olfaction is accompanied by the rise to power of vision, particularly of stereoscopic vision. This is seen in the change from lateral placement of the eyes to a frontal positioning which permits an increase in the overlap of visual fields. This increase in the binocular segment correlates in living primates with the proportion of uncrossed fibres in the optic chiasm (see Chapter 2 of this volume). An insectivore such as the tree shrew has laterally implanted eyes and approximately 10 per cent of uncrossed fibres in the chiasm. This contrasts with prosimians such as the galago and the loris, both of which have more frontally placed eyes and also have 40–50 per cent of uncrossed fibres in the chiasm. Stephan (1969) has explained the changes in the relative volume of the visual cortex and the lateral geniculate bodies for prosimians, simians and anthropoids. As can be seen in Figure 6.4 the amount of visual (striate) cortex increases in prosimians relative to lepilemur standard which was used in the absence of data from insectivores. The same is true for simians, whereas for anthropoid apes and man the striate cortex forms a lower proportion of total cortex. This could suggest that the growth of other cortical areas have increased their share of the neocortex at the expense of the visual cortex. None the less, it is again a

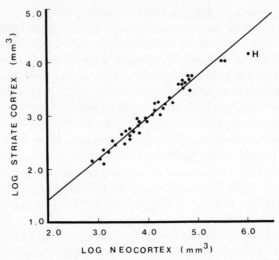

Fig. 6.4   Relationship between volume of striate cortex and volume of total neocortex in prosimians, monkeys and anthropoid apes, including man (H). From Passingham and Ettlinger 1974.

similar picture, in that the amount of visual cortex is determined directly by the changes in brain size.

From what has been considered so far it would appear as though the neocortex is the sole beneficiary of the increase in relative brain size. The evidence is clear that the limbic structures also increase during evolution relative to brain size. Stephan et al. (1970) have reported that the changes in the size of hippocampus from insectivores to prosimians to anthropoids are closely related to changes in total brain weight (see Figure 6.5).

Sacher (1970) has analysed formally the relations between brain size and the relative volumes of the various structures of the brain in insectivores and primates. In agreement with much of what has been covered so far, his essential finding was that overall brain size can be used to estimate the size of most parts of the brain. The correlation between brain size and cerebellum was 0·996; brain size and neocortex was 0·989; and for brain size and the diencephalon was 0·995. The correlation between brain size and body weight was less perfect at 0·945; and a similar value of 0·941 was found for the correlation with paleocortex. It was only the olfactory bulb that was not highly correlated with brain size, where a value of 0·350 was obtained. It should be noted that what this means is that although the olfactory bulbs increase in size in absolute terms, they do not increase in the same relative proportion to brain size as do the other parts of the brain. It would appear therefore, that the major change in evolution is a progressive increase in the relative brain size of the whole brain, rather than in any particular brain structure such as neocortex.

Thus no marked differences have emerged in the changes in the gross morphology of the mammalian brain during evolution other than an increase in cerebral mass. It is therefore logical to consider whether there are any differences in the density of packing of the neurons in the brains of different animals. If the cell density packing factor per unit volume of brain is constant in simple and complex brains, this would suggest that differences in encephalization derive essentially from variations in the number of cells. The earliest estimates of cell density come from Mayer (1912) who showed that cell

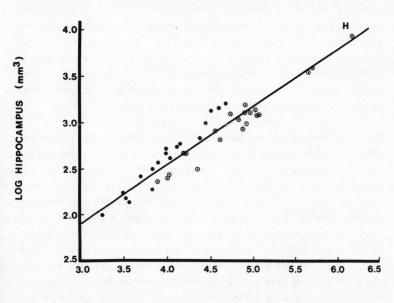

Fig. 6.5   Relationship between volume of hippocampus and brain weight in prosimians (single dots), primates and anthropoid apes (circled dots) and man (H). From Passingham and Ettlinger 1974.

density decreased as cortical volume increased. This was replicated by Shariff (1953) using the same prosimian, simian and anthropoid series of animals. Again cell density both for sensory or association cortex was found to decrease as the brain size increased. Similarly Chow et al. (1950) and Tower (1954) found that this inverse relationship between cell packing density and brain size was not peculiar to primates but was characteristic of the entire mammalian series. For example the number of cells per 0·001 mm³ varied from 950 for mouse, 502 for rat, 302 for rabbit, 242 for cat, 204 for dog, 215 for monkey, 105 for man and 68 for the elephant. It should be stressed that large brains coincide with low cell density packing *independently* of the degree of encephalization.

Bok (1959) examined the possibility that the low neuron density packing factor associated with larger brains would permit more elaborate dendritic branching and glial cell distribution in the greater space between neurons. Thus the true significance of the lower cell density of big brains would be to enable greater connectivity between neurons. Bok compared homologous neurons over a series of rodents. He measured the lengths of dendritic trees for cells in the cortex of a mouse, rat, guinea-pig and rabbit and reported that as the neuron density diminished, the lengths of dendritic arborization increased. Jerison (1973) interprets this finding as evidence for greater circuit complexity and information handling capability.

Although this view is attractive for psychological theories, it is based on very uncertain anatomical foundations. First, the decrease in neuron packing density is associated with absolute brain size and not relative brain size. Thus the chimpanzee with a brain weight of 440 gms has a packing density value of 174 cells for 0·001 mm³ (Shariff, 1953), and the ox with a brain of 493 gms has the same packing density value of 174 cells per 0·001 mm³ (Chow et al. 1950). This is despite the enormous difference both in relative brain size for the two animals and in intellect! Secondly, Sholl (1950) drew attention to the dramatic variation of the density packing factor in the same animal, both within the same as well as different regions of the cortex, dependent on the cortical depth. Further, given the fact that cell size also changes due to brain size, cortical region and depth, it is obvious that this type of cytoarchitectonic enquiry is inherently unreliable and selective.

Thus the most striking change during the evolution of the nervous system is the increase in the gross brain size or mass of cells. The suggestion by Bok (1959) and Jerison (1973) that larger and more encephalized brains have qualitative differences in their connectivity options was not found to be convincing. The changes in the neuronal density packing factor between species was no greater than within a species. Thus there is every reason to agree with Lashley (1949) when he said: 'The only neurological character for which a correlation with behavioural capacity in different animals is supported by significant evidence is the total mass of tissue, or rather, the index of cephalization, measured by the ratio of brain to total body weight, which seems to represent the amount of tissue in excess of that required for transmitting impulses to and from the integrative centers.'

Encephalization, the emergence of cortex, and the evolution of intelligence

As the brain develops in size and complexity in the phylogenetic series from fish to man, it has generally been concluded that functions that were originally controlled by lower systems were taken over by the cerebrum. This progressive shift of dominance to the higher centres was termed encephalization of function and has traditionally been a major principle in the evolution of the brain. The concept of encephalization has been used to characterize most of the functions of the brain including motor activity, sensory discrimination and learning. Marquis (1935), for instance, claimed that in the absence of a cerebrum or cortex, fish and birds show no signs of motor disturbance; whereas after decortication the rat, cat and dog show increasing signs of motor impairment. The decorticate monkey is the most severely impaired, in that it is completely unable to walk. Marquis proposed a similar trend in the case of vision. Following decerebration there is no apparent impairment of vision in fish, and little change in the bird. The decorticate rat is impaired with pattern vision, but can still distinguish between brightness, position and distance of objects. The cat, dog and monkey retain only brightness perception, whereas man was said to become completely blind. A similar trend has also been claimed for the effect of decortication on learning (see Chapter 7 of this volume).

Two points need to be made concerning this view of functional encephalization. First, it has only ever had heuristic value for mammalian development; it has been misleading with regard to avian evolution. Second, the principle of encephalization is no longer compatible with contemporary research on the effects of cortical lesions in mammals (Weiskrantz, 1961). Nowadays the notion that a function remains constant while changing its cerebral machinery as one moves through the mammalian series is rejected. Instead it is believed that a function such as vision is processed somewhat differently in different species. For example, form vision in the rat tends to involve local flux analysis in preference to more articulate feature extraction such as orientation or pattern-information. In the primate not only would the latter analyses have priority, but they would also be combined with information about colour and stereoscopic disparity. Thus a simple visual discrimination task would be analysed by different brains in very different ways, using very different neural circuits or computational routines.

Faced with the progressive evolution of the brain, a major concern of the comparative psychologist and physiologist has been to evaluate the significance and these changes for the relative intelligence of the various species. This has proved to be a difficult task for several reasons. First, it assumes a simple relationship between learning and intelligence. Second, valid comparisons of learning ability are difficult to make in view of the very great sensori-motor differences that exist between species. For example the 'control systems' used by a rat and a monkey in a two-choice visual discrimination task are profoundly different. The rat must use vision both to identify the correct pattern (targeting) and to steer itself to the target location (visual guidance) to make a choice response. The monkey by contrast only needs vision for visual targeting. No visual guidance is required as it can use kinaesthesis to reach with a hand to make a choice. An additional problem is variation in motivation between species where there are difficulties in obtaining comparable incentive-reward conditions for different animals. Where differences in metabolic rate exist, as between a rat and a lizard, the problems are formidable. The use of electric shock can be advantageous for motivating an animal such as a rat, but devastating for a tree shrew. From this point of view it is evident that any learning differences between species could always be argued to result from motivational differences. Finally the presence of species' typical behaviours can either facilitate learning or retard it, dependent on the form of interaction between the behaviour and the task. For example, operant learning in birds is maximized if they are required to peck at a key, but it is severely limited if they are asked to bar press with their feet.

In general, where cross-species comparisons of learning ability are made, the acquisition rates are similar for a wide variety of animals (Razran, 1933). Pavlovian conditioning of a dorsal-fin response in fish and leg-flexion in both pigeon and sheep to an auditory signal, for example, all required a similar number of trials. It should be mentioned that had these findings provided evidence that learning rates differed between animals, this would not be attributable to species differences in learning ability. It would merely reflect the effect of procedural differences on acquisition rate. Indeed it is questionable whether any quantitative differences in the learning of a task could ever be attributed to true learning differences between species (for a detailed consideration of the effect of procedural variations on Pavlovian conditioning, see Brookshire, 1970). Considering instrumental learning similar results have been found. Bitterman (1960) reported that the rate of learning in a maze is identical for the bird, rat and monkey. Indeed Lashley (1929) also reported rats and humans to be equally proficient with respect to maze learning. These findings endorse Lashley's comment:

> The comparative study of learning in different animals gives little evidence that evolution has brought any change in the rate of formation of simpler habits. On the other hand, there is a fairly consistent rise in the limits of training and in the formation of complex habits with ascent in the phylogenetic scale.

The lack of success in finding cross-species differences for learning is perhaps due to the elementary nature of the tasks used. If this is the case then it is unlikely that differences in intelligence between species would emerge in terms of the speed of data processing or rate of acquisition. In view of the fact that the principal evolutionary change in the brain is an increase in size, it is more reasonable to expect differences in adjustment to more complex or abstract data processing problems.

It has been traditional to consider that the frontal association cortex is in some sense intimately associated with intelligence or abstract thought and is one of the characteristics separating man from beast. It is certainly true that the frontal cortex increases relative to total cortex throughout the mammalian series. The amount of frontal cortex in cat is 3 per cent of the total cortex; in dog the proportion increases to 9 per cent; it is 12 per cent for the macaque, 15 per cent in chimpanzee, and 24 per cent in man (Blinkov and Glazer, 1968).

Jacobsen (1935) suggested that the frontal lobes were responsible for immediate memory. He found that after the removal of the prefrontal areas of cortex, monkeys were unable to perform a task involving a delay of several seconds before responding to a stimulus. Typically in these delayed-response problems the animal is given a cue as to the location of a reward (e.g. the placing of a peanut under one of two cups in front of the animal). It is then restrained for a variable delay time, and then tested to see if it remembers which choice to make. Hunter (1913) originally standardized this behavioural test as a measure of symbolic or ideational processes in animals.

Following Jacobsen's discovery that the ability to make a delayed response is dependent on the integrity of the frontal lobes, comparative psychologists attempted to use it to differentiate species according to their encephalization level. This resulted in a substantial body of research which did not reveal any consistent trend. Maier and Schneirla (1964) pointed out that not only was the variability within any species greater than the differences between them, but that such results were highly subject to procedural bias. They showed that every species studied could delay successfully for hours if tested with distinctly different response alternatives, and conversely that no species could delay its response when the alternatives lacked distinctiveness. Since that time it has been shown that success with the delayed response is highly dependent upon attention during the initial observing response (Fletcher, 1965). Other determining factors of success or failure are: degree of motivation, size of reward, body orientation during the delay period, intertrial interval, number of daily trials, etc. When these factors are considered, it is obvious that they will always overshadow any potential interspecies differences. Some standardization may be possible for related species, but this will not be feasible where there are considerable differences between species, e.g. carnivores compared to primates.

The possibility that differences exist between species in the ability 'to learn how to learn' has been investigated using learning sets and probability learning tasks. Typically a learning set involves a two-choice discrimination for either a spatial or a visual task. Following training for a fixed number of trials or to some performance criterion, the animal is then required to reverse the discrimination. After receiving the same number of trials or reaching the same criterion as before, the problem is reversed again and so on. Monkeys, rats and pigeons trained in this manner normally show a steady and progressive improvement with successive reversals of either a spatial or a visual task. Gradually each reversal is obtained more rapidly and with fewer errors as the animal learns to learn. A fish shows no such improvement for either the spatial or visual tasks. The turtle, on the other hand, showed no learning set for visual reversals, but did show some savings for spatial reversals where no savings are seen even after 14 reversals. (Bitterman, 1968)

Species differences have also been claimed for probability learning tasks. In a two-choice discrimination, alternative A would be rewarded randomly for 70 per cent of the trials and alternative B for the remaining 30 per cent of trials. A monkey or a rat in such a situation 'maximizes' its choice by selecting the most probable stimulus on almost all trials. By contrast fish and turtles demonstrate a different strategy where they 'match' the reward possibilities. That is, the distribution of choices made approximates the distribution of rewards without any obvious sequential response patterning. However these different choice strategies can be determined by situational and procedural factors more often than by species differences.

Considering the research on learning set, great caution has to be exercised (see also Chapter 7 of this volume). In common with all behavioural measures of learning, variation due to procedural differences is much greater than species differences. For example Hayes et al. (1953) found that a chimpanzee, given learning set training with 2 trials per problem, remained at chance levels of performance for 300 problems. There was a dramatic improvement with 10 trials per problem where *intraproblem* learning was possible. Many other factors affect learning set performance. The discriminability of stimuli used is a crucial determinent of learning. Interference between problems can retard acquisition. Stereometric stimuli facilitate learning set acquisition, and planometric displays retard it. The amount and type of reward have potent effects on some species and not others. Drive effects similarly differ between species. Thus it would appear that any quantification of species differences with respect to learning set or probability learning is made virtually meaningless because learning depends on an *adventitious* interaction of many variables. Furthermore the exact mode of action of these variables is not known across species.

It is also true to say that these difficulties apply equally well when we study the effect of brain lesions on learning. The effect of any lesion is most likely to alter the 'tuning' of the animal to the experimental procedure rather than to affect directly any brain mechanism responsible for learning *per se*.

Conclusions

The present survey has considered the general problem of evaluating the significance of changes in brain size and their potential relationship to intelligence. Although brain size can vary enormously in any vertebrate species, the evidence from man shows this to have no significance as far as intelligence is concerned. Thus it was argued that to evaluate changes in brain size is only meaningful within the broad context of vertebrate development. Within that conceptual framework it was seen that 'lower' vertebrates such as fish and reptiles have evolved brains which have an exact allometric relationship to the requirements of their body size, in the same manner as their other internal organs such as the heart or the liver. Birds and mammals were found to have evolved enlarged brains, in excess of this body size factor. Furthermore it was noted that this development in brain size is not explicable in terms of the traditional theory of encephalization (see Chapter 2 of this volume). Instead it was seen that there is a uniform enlargement of all brain structures with the exception of the olfactory bulbs.

Comparative studies of simple learning were seen to have no relation to brain size or development. Indeed the work of Kandel (1967) and Krasne (1973) has not only shown that invertebrates have basic learning abilities, but has already made substantial progress in elucidating the neural networks involved. From many points of view it would seem that the notion that species-related learning characteristics is a dated and archaic position (see also Chapter 7 of this volume). Indeed the anthropomorphic notion of a hierarchy of species (e.g. Bitterman, 1968) with a correlated hierarchy of intellectual skills is not supported by evidence. Historically this view was derived from the classical theory of encephalization of function. Thus with the demise of that principle only intellectual inertia remains to support it.

Certainly from an evolutionary viewpoint there is no scale that phylogenetically ranks species according to their varying degrees of success in approximating primates and man. In evolution there was the adaptive radiation of species into many different ecological niches. Survival demands requiring enlargement of the brain occurred rarely and always in relation to particular niches. This has been an episodic and not a continuous process.

From this point of view the relationship between brain size and intelligence can be restated. If the neuron can be regarded as the 'atomic' unit of function in the nervous system, then the 'molecular' unit of information processing is the 'miniature nervous system' (mns). Such cell configurations have only recently been isolated (Bullock, 1967), but their widespread occurrence qualifies them to be considered as fundamental building blocks in neural evolution. They operate as a prewired neural assembly, where individual cells are configured to execute fairly complex transactions analogous to an integrated circuit (ic) chip. For example, one neuron in an mns may always be excited or inhibited when a second neuron is activated; or the pattern of excitation-inhibition may change in consistent modes in response to being driven by the second neuron. What is most important is that the work of aplysia and crayfish shows that simple forms of learning such as habituation and conditioning occur in these neural units.

Considering the mns as a data processing unit in the brain enables one to speculate on the function of brain size. The increase in the number of such units is perhaps analogous to core storage in a computer. The greater the information storage capacity, the greater the flexibility there is in generating data-processing programmes with optional subroutines. This permits the same data to be handled in different ways in different circumstances; or different data to be analysed as having the same meaning. Thus bigger brains do not need to learn differently; they can simply generate longer data control programmes with option flexibility for changes in context or circumstance. Perhaps this is part of what we mean by intelligence.

References

Bitterman, M. E. (1960) Toward a comparative psychology of learning. *American Psychologist 15*: 704–12.

Bitterman, M. E. (1968) Phyletic differences in learning. In N. S. Endler, L. R. Boulter and H. Osser (eds) *Contemporary Issues in Developmental Psychology*. New York: Holt, Rinehart & Winston, 77–94.

Blinkov, S. M. and Glazer, I. I. (1968) *The Human Brain: A quantitative handbook*. New York: Basic Books and Plenum Press.

Bok, S. T. (1959) *Histonomy of the Cerebral Cortex*. Princeton, N.J.: Van Nostrand-Reinhold.

Brookshire, K. H. (1970) Comparative psychology of learning. In M. H. Marc (ed. *Learning: Interactions*. London: Macmillan, 290–364.

Bullock, T. H. (1967) Simple systems for the study of learning mechanisms. In F. O. Schmitt et al. (eds) *Neuroscience Research Summaries*, Vol. 2. Cambridge, Mass.: MIT Press, 203–327.

Chow, K. L., Blum, J. S. and Blum, K. A. (1950) Cell ratios in the thalamocortical visual system of macaca mulatta. *Journal of Comparative Neurology 92* (2): 227–39.

Crile, G. W. and Quiring, D. P. (1940) A record of the body weights and certain organs and gland weights of 3690 animals. *Ohio Journal of Science 40* (5): 219–59.

Dubois, E. (1897) Sur le rapport du poids de l'encéphale avec la grandeur du corps chez les mammifères. *Bulletin de la société d'anthropologie de Paris 8*: 337–76.

Elias, H. and Schwartz, D. (1969) Surface areas of the cerebral cortex of mammals determined by stereological methods. *Science 166*: 111–13.

Fletcher, H. J. (1965) The delayed response problem. In A. M. Schrier, H. E. Harlow and F. Stollnitz (eds) *Behavior of Non-human Primates*, Vol. 1, New York: Academic Press, 129–65.

Harman, P. J. L. (1957) Paleoneurologic, neoneurologic and ontogenetic aspects of brain phylogeny. James Arthur lecture on the evolution of the human brain. American Museum of Natural History, New York.

Hunter, W. S. (1913) The delayed reaction in animals and children. *Behavioural Monograph 2* (1) (Serial No. 6).

Hayes, K. J., Thompson, R. and Hayes, C. (1953) Discrimination learning set in chimpanzees. *Journal of Comparative and Physiological Psychology 46*: 99–112.

Jacobsen, C. F. (1935) Functions of the frontal association area in primates. *Arch. Neurol. Psychiat. 33*: 558–69.

Jerison, H. J. (1973) *Evolution of Intelligence*. New York: Academic Press.

Kandel, E. R. (1967) An invertebrate system for the cellular analysis of simple behaviors and their modifications. In F. O. Schmidt and F. C. Worden (eds) *The Neurosciences: Third Study Program*. Cambridge, Mass.: MIT Press, 347–70.

Krasne, F. B. (1973) Learning in crustacea. In W. C. Corning, J. A. Dyal and A. O. D. Willows (eds) *Invertebrate Learning, 2*. New York: Plenum Press.

Lashley, K. S. (1929) Nervous mechanisms in learning. In C. Murchison (ed.) *The Foundations of Experimental Psychology*. Worcester, Mass.: Clark University Press, 524–63.

Lashley, K. S. (1949) Persistent problems in the evolution of mind. *Quarterly Review of Biology 24*: 28–42.

Leboucq, G. (1929) Le rapport entre le poids et la surface de l'hemisphere cerebrale chez l'homme et les singes. *Mem. Acad. Roy. Belg. 10*: 55–72.

Maier, N. R. F. and Schnierla, T. C. (1964) *Principles of Animal Psychology* (2nd edn). New York: Dover.

Marquis, D. G. (1935) Phylogenetic interpretation of the functions of the visual cortex. *Arch. Neurol. Psychiat. 33*: 807–15.

Mayer, O. (1912) Given in Blinkov and Glazer (1968), p. 402.

Muhlman, L. (1957) Given in Blinkov and Glazer (1968), p. 334.

Passingham, R. E. and Ettlinger, G. (1974) A comparison of cortical functions in man and other primates. *International Review of Neurobiology 16*: 233–99.

Penrose, L. (1949) *The Biology of the Mental Defective*. London: Methuen.

Quiring, D. P. (1941) The scale of being according to the power formula. *Growth 5*: 301–27.

Radinsky, L. (1975) Primate brain evolution. *American Scientist 63*: 6, 656–63.

Razran, G. H. S. (1933) Conditioned responses in animals other than dogs. *Psychological Bulletin 30*: 261–324.

Sacher, G. A. (1970) Allometric and factorial analyses of brain structure in insectivores and primates. In C. R. Noback and W. Montagna (eds) *The Primate Brain*, Vol. 1. New York: Appleton Century Crofts, 245–87.

Scholl, D. A. (1948) The quantitative investigation of the vertebrate brain and the applicability of allometric formulae to its study. *Proc. Roy. Soc., Ser. B. 135*: 243–58.

Scholl, D. A. (1956) *The Organization of the Cerebral Cortex*. London: Methuen.

Shariff, G. A. (1953) Cell counts in the primate cerebral cortex. *Journal of Comparative Neurology 98*: 381–400.

Snell, O. (1891) Die abhangigkeit des Hirngewichtes von dem Korpergewicht und den geistigen Fahigkeitern. *Arch. Psychiat. Nervenkz.* 23: 436–46.

Stephan, H. (1969) Quantitative investigations on visual structures in primate brains. Proc. 2nd Int. Cong. Primat. 3: 34–42. Basel/N.Y. Karger.

Stephan, H. and Andy, O. J. (1969) Quantitative comparative neuroanatomy of primates: an attempt at a phyletic interpretation. *Annals of the N.Y. Academy of Science 167*: 370–87.

Stephan, H., Bauchot, R. and Andy, O. J. (1970) Data on size of the brain and of various brain parts in insectivores and primates. In C. R. Noback and W. Montagna (eds) *The Primate Brain*, Vol. 1. New York: Appleton Century Crofts, 289–97.

Tower, D. B. (1954) Structural and functional organization of mammalian cerebral cortex; the correlation of neurone density with brain size. *Journal of Comparative Neurology 101*: 19–51.

von Bonin, G. (1937) Brain weight and body weight in mammals. *Journal of General Psychology 16*: 379–89.

Weiskrantz, L. (1961) Encephalization and the scotoma. In W. H. Thorpe and O. L. Zangwill (eds) *Current Problems in Animal Behaviour*. Cambridge University Press, 30–98.

7 Cerebral cortex and adaptive behaviour

David A. Oakley

Introduction

One of the most striking changes in the evolution of mammals from an ancestral reptilian stock has been the expansion of neocortical tissue over the surface of the cerebral hemispheres (see Chapters 2 and 6 of this volume). In so far as behaviour can be said to have increased in its range and effectiveness during the same evolutionary process it is tempting to conclude that the expansion of both neocortex and of behavioural horizons are linked. As if to underline this conclusion, in man the richly folded neocortex represents almost the entire visible surface of the intact brain and is assumed to be the anatomical feature above all others which accounts for his intellectual uniqueness. This is all very well at an intuitive level but 'adaptive behaviour', 'behavioural horizons' and 'intellectual uniqueness' are vague terms and it is necessary to specify just which abilities are being equated with neocortical tissue before any systematic analysis can begin. The traditional first contender is the ability to learn from past and present experience and to utilize that learning in controlling behaviour on future occasions.

Neocortex and learning

Comparative studies

Though the idea that learning depends on neocortex has a long history there is one serious objection to it, namely that comparative learning studies show that neocortex is manifestly *not* a prerequisite for learning. Learning represents a fine-tuner to the evolutionary process whereby the individual organism can adapt its behaviour to the environment during its lifetime within the broad guidelines given by hereditary mechanisms (see Chapters 1 and 3 of this volume and Plotkin and Odling-Smee, 1979). Purely genetic processes are limited in their ability to predict future environmental changes and so cannot provide pre-wired responses for every contingency. Thus it is likely that the ability to learn emerged early in evolutionary history, long before the evolution of neocortex, to enhance the biological fitness of individuals. Fish, for example, do not possess neocortex at all and yet have been found to learn in simple situations at about the same rate as other vertebrates and may even be quicker than monkeys on some problems (Warren, 1974). Birds, in which neocortex is sparse or absent, have provided, via the pigeon, a standard subject for learning studies in psychology laboratories and as a class can out-perform some mammals in a variety of complex learning problems (Stettner and Matyniak, 1968). It is apparently not even necessary to be a vertebrate to learn and many studies have claimed to demonstrate learning in invertebrates from the single-celled paramecium to the highly complex octopus (McConnell and Jacobson, 1974). Nor, for that matter, is it necessary to be an animal. A number of well-controlled studies seem to indicate simple learning capacities in the sensitive plant, *Mimosa pudica* (Sanberg, 1976).

Encephalization of learning

It is clear then that the sort of cellular plasticity required to mediate learning is possible in tissues other than neocortex. In the case of mammals, however, neocortex *is* present and becomes increasingly well developed in certain mammalian lines. Is it possible that as this newer tissue evolved it took over functions, including the ability to learn, from the older parts of the brain? This is the once-popular notion of encephalization, or corticalization, of function which would see neocortex in this case taking over the role of learning, leaving subcortex to specialize in the control of more reflexive responses aimed at regulating the internal state of the organism (see also Chapters 2 and 6 of this volume). More recently the idea that functions migrate upwards in this fashion during evolution has been criticized on both factual and theoretical grounds (Jerison, 1973 and Weiskrantz, 1977). In particular, given the usual conservatism of the evolutionary process it would be surprising if newer structures evolved to subserve functions already carried out by existing structures. Nevertheless, the assumption of encephalization shaped many early views of brain and behaviour and the generally corticocentric view of the brain which it fostered has proved highly resistant to change. A number of early writers were thus able to equate neocortex with learning ability within the theoretical framework of encephalization and so avoided criticisms which might otherwise have been advanced on the basis of comparative studies of learning ability.

Pavlovian conditioning and instrumental learning

Pavlov (1927) concluded on the basis of studies with dogs which had had neocortex surgically removed (neodecorticated – see Figure 7.1) that this part of the mammalian brain was essential for learning to take place. He drew this conclusion 'with the utmost reserve' though many of his students took the more extreme view that learning could not, by definition, occur in the absence of neocortex. Pavlov's account of conditioning assumed that associations were formed in neocortex between the analyser for one stimulus, the conditional stimulus (CS), and the analyser for a second stimulus, the unconditional stimulus (US). The procedural and behavioural differences between Pavlovian conditioning and instrumental learning are important to what follows and a detailed account of them can be found in Mackintosh (1974). In time it became clear that mammals without neocortex could in fact learn in Pavlovian conditioning situations and neodecorticated dogs were shown to acquire diffuse conditional responses (CRs) to acoustic, thermal and tactile CSs when these stimuli were paired with shock as the US (e.g. Girden et al., 1936). More recently, totally neodecorticated rabbits have been found to acquire finely controlled nictitating membrane (third eyelid) responses to both tone and light CSs, using cheek shock as the US. These animals were

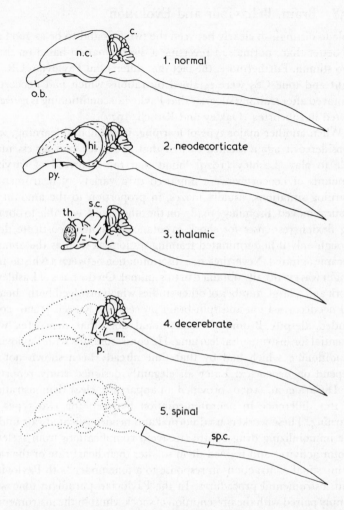

Fig. 7.1 This figure shows a normal rabbit brain and spinal cord and the four stages of nervous system reduction described in the text. If recent specializations are ignored the neodecorticated rabbit brain approximates that of a primitive reptile in terms of the gross anatomical structures present. Damaged brain tissue in parts 2 and 3 of the figure is shown by irregular dashes. Dotted outlines in parts 4 and 5 indicate that these preparations are usually produced by transecting the brain rather than by removing the more rostral structures completely. Only the isolated part of the brain below the cut is tested. Abbreviations: c. = cerebellum; hi. = hippocampus; m. = medulla; n.c. = neocortex; o.b. = olfactory bulb; p. = pons; py. = pyriform cortex; s.c. = superior colliculus; sp.c. = spinal cord; th. = thalamus (see also Chapter 2 of this volume).

able to distinguish clearly between the two CSs and to be as good as, or better than, normals at reversing a discrimination based on these two stimuli. Furthermore, the fact that differential Pavlovian CRs to light and tone CSs were retained by rabbits which had neocortex removed after training suggests that Pavlovian conditioning is *normally* stored in subcortex (Oakley and Russell, 1977).

When another major type of learning, instrumental learning, was considered it again seemed at first that neocortex had an essential role to play. Lashley (1929) found that rats deprived of varying amounts of neocortex were impaired in a variety of instrumental learning situations, usually mazes, in proportion to the amount of tissue removed. Bromiley (1948), on the other hand, was able to obtain leg flexion responses for shock avoidance in a neodecorticate dog, though only if he terminated training sessions as soon as the animal became agitated. Nevertheless, a discrimination between a whistle and a light was eventually obtained in this animal. On the basis of Lashley's work and a large number of other studies which involved both chemical neodecortication and split-brain procedures, Russell (1966) concluded, despite Bromiley's exceptional dog, that neocortex was essential for instrumental learning. He contrasted this with Pavlovian conditioning which had by that time already been shown not to depend on neocortex. Later an elegantly designed study reported by DiCara et al. (1970) provided an apparently clear demonstration of this difference in neural mediation between the two types of learning. These workers used normal and neodecorticated rats under the immobilizing drug curare (to avoid complications from skeletal motor activity) and trained them to alter their heart rate or the rate of intestinal contractions in response to a tone under both Pavlovian and instrumental procedures. In the Pavlovian paradigm tone was simply paired with the presentation of shock whilst in the instrumental procedure the animal could avoid the shock by altering its heart or intestinal responses appropriately. The sensory and motor requirements were identical in both Pavlovian and instrumental conditions and normal rats learned to respond under both procedures. Neodecorticated rats, however, formed Pavlovian CRs but did not learn to alter these same responses to avoid shock under the instrumental training condition.

Since the DiCara et al. study contradictory data have emerged and neodecorticated rabbits have been shown to be capable of working for food reward in a modified Skinner box (Oakley, 1971; Oakley and

Russell, 1978). This particular instrumental response was acquired a little more slowly by the neodecorticates than the normal animals and was rather less efficiently performed. With a pretraining programme which directed the animals' attention to the relevant parts of the apparatus, however, the neodecorticates became far more efficient and were able to perform effectively on reinforcement schedules which required as many as 60 treadle presses for each reinforcement pellet(a Fixed Ratio 60 or FR60 schedule) (Oakley, 1978). This has since been repeated in neodecorticated rats and represents quite an impressive performance in what is usually considered to be an instrumental learning situation.

One question which these recent studies raise is why the earlier studies obtained poor, or even no, instrumental learning in the absence of neocortex. One possible reason is the fact that the earlier studies used shock avoidance procedures. An experiment I have recently completed with neodecorticated and normal rats showed that the neodecorticates could learn to run along an alleyway for food as well as normal animals but could not learn to run in the same alleyway to avoid shock. This failure to perform adaptively in the presence of foot shock was seen even if the animals had already learned with food reward to traverse the alleyway at speeds which would ensure that they avoided shock completely. Bromiley (1948) had noted that his neodecorticated dog became more than normally agitated if it received shock and the rats in the alleyway study similarly became disturbed and refused to run once they encountered the first shock, even though they received foot shock for longer by so doing. It could be then that the early studies were measuring not so much an inability to learn but a tendency on the part of neodecorticates to become hyperemotional in the presence of painful stimuli. The classic studies of Bard and Mountcastle (1948) showed in fact that if neocortex alone was removed in cats the animal became abnormally placid. If the lesion extended just outside neocortex a very different picture emerged in which even mildly unpleasant stimuli evoked a rage response out of all proportion to the stimulus. In my own studies as well as those of Bromiley (1948) and DiCara et al. (1970) the lesions extended slightly beyond the strict limits of neocortex and so were likely on Bard and Mountcastle's evidence to produce animals which could be abnormally disturbed by noxious stimuli. Whilst much work remains to be done it seems reasonable to conclude for the moment that learning is possible using instrumental procedures in neodecorticated animals provided they are not exposed to aversive stimulation during training. It is worth remembering though that shock is a perfectly adequate US for Pavlovian conditioning in neodecorticates (see above).

Learning theorists would perhaps wish to make one further reservation at this point. Namely, that whilst the learning situations I have just been describing are by traditional definitions instrumental, there is currently considerable debate as to the extent to which they contain, or may even be completely explained on the basis of, covert Pavlovian conditioning (see Schwartz and Gamzu, 1977). It is not appropriate to enter a discussion of this question here except perhaps to note that any suggestion that so-called instrumental learning may be explained by Pavlovian mechanisms (autoshaping or sign tracking: the tendency of animals to explore stimuli which predict reward) applies to normals as well as to neodecorticates. The possibility that the decorticates are solving the 'instrumental' problem one way and the normals another cannot be dismissed however. It is certainly true on the present evidence that neodecortication makes acquisition in traditionally defined instrumental situations more difficult, whereas traditional Pavlovian conditioning is little if at all affected by the same lesion. The neodecorticate's difficulty in the instrumental situation seems to lie, however, in defining the salient features of its environment rather than in learning the relationship between them and reinforcement.

Learning in thalamic, decerebrate and spinal preparations

If neocortex is not essential for learning in the mammalian brain it is interesting to consider briefly just how much, or how little, of such brains *is* required for learning to take place (see review by Berlucchi and Buchtel, 1975). The next stage of brain reduction from neodecortication involves the removal of the other major telencephalic structures – limbic cortex, hippocampus and basal ganglia – leaving a so-called thalamic preparation; the thalamus being the most rostral structure remaining intact (see Figure 7.1). There is little doubt that thalamic animals can learn Pavlovian responses and recent studies of eyeblink conditioning in thalamic cats have produced normal looking acquisition, extinction, differentiation and reversal data using both auditory and visual CSs. Instrumental learning has been less frequently documented in thalmic preparations but Huston and

Borbély (1974), using rats, found that their thalamic animals would acquire a variety of responses, such as head turning, wall climbing, tail raising or even walking backwards, if these behaviours were rewarded with electrical stimulation of a 'pleasure' site in the hypothalamus. In a similar fashion essentially thalamic cats would learn a T-maze discrimination though, interestingly enough in the light of the neodecortication findings, only for food reward. Shock caused maladaptive freezing reactions and prevented learning (Bjursten et al., 1976). Despite its popularity as a preparation with neurophysiologists the decerebrated mammal, that is one with all tissue above the midbrain either removed completely or surgically isolated (see Figure 7.1), has received rather less attention from those concerned with learning. Convincing evidence has been obtained, however, that Pavlovian conditioning is possible and Norman et al. (1977), for example, found normal patterns of eyeblink conditioning, including tone differentiation and reversal, in decerebrate cats.

Intuitively the spinal cord is the least likely part of the central nervous system in which learning would be expected. It is the part most likely to have surrendered its plasticity to higher structures if the theory of encephalization of function has any validity. It is commonly depicted as a bundle of fibres passing information to and from the brain with some provision for pre-wired, reflexive responses, albeit of some complexity, concerned with posture and defence. It is perhaps surprising then that the spinal preparation – one with the spinal cord isolated from the rest of the brain (see Figure 7.1) – has recieved rather a lot of attention over the years from researchers interested in the neural substrata of learning (see Buchwald and Brown, 1973). It is less surprising to find that their repeated claims to have found evidence of learning in the spinal cord have met with considerable scepticism, due in part to the difficulty of finding a convincing learning situation suited to the spinal cord's limited sensory (touch) and motor (leg flexion, muscle twitch) capacities. Pavlovian conditioning in the cat spinal cord using direct sensory nerve stimulation as the CS, stimulation of another nerve as the US, and recording direct muscle activity as both the unconditional response (UR) and the CR has now been demonstrated in experimental designs which control for non-learning effects such as sensitization (e.g. Light and Durkovic, 1977).

Instrumental learning has also been demonstrated recently in spinal rats under similarly carefully controlled conditions. Chopin and

Buerger (1975) suspended pairs of spinal rats over a saline bath, designated one rat of each pair as the experimental animal and the other served as a yoked control. Whenever the experimental animal dipped its hind leg into the liquid both animals recieved a direct electric shock to the leg. Shock was terminated for both animals when the experimental animal raised its leg. The yoked animal thus received exactly the same shocks as the experimental animal but, unlike the experimental animal, it received them independently of its leg position. The experimental animals but not the yoked controls learned to keep their legs out of the liquid to avoid shock. It was also possible in this study to shape the experimental animals' leg response to ever greater flexion by slowly raising the level of the liquid as training progressed.

Habituation

I have concentrated on Pavlovian conditioning and instrumental learning in the above discussion at the expense of a third major category of learning: habituation (the tendency of organisms to cease responding to repetitive and unimportant stimuli). In fact habituation has generally been regarded as so fundamental a process that the fact it has been demonstrated in all animals and in all' of the reduced nervous systems shown in Figure 7.1 has been readily accepted (see Buchwald and Brown, 1973; Russell 1966; Tighe and Leaton, 1976).

Conclusions

The conclusion that the entire mammalian central nervous system has retained sufficiently plasticity to mediate habituation, Pavlovian conditioning and instrumental learning seems inescapable. There is no evidence that function, at least at the level of simple learning, has been encephalized and consequently little basis for equating neo-cortex, or indeed any other part of the central nervous system, exclusively with any one type of learning in mammals. There is also very little evidence so far, either anatomical or phylogenetic, to sustain the common, though usually implicit, ranking of types of learning which holds that habituation is simplest or 'most primitive', that Pavlovian conditioning is one stage more complex or 'more evolved', and that instrumental learning is the most complex or 'highest'. All types of animal and all levels of the mammalian nervous system are able to handle all three categories of learning. This might favour the view that learning *per se* is not a 'higher' process but rather a basic activity requiring at most only a small number of neurones in the form of micro-processing units or 'miniature nervous systems' to carry it out in its three basic paradigmatic versions. Behavioural capacity or intelligence may then be a function of the number and variety of such micro-processors present (see Jerison, 1973, and Chapter 6 of this volume).

Neocortex and learning sets

The simple ability to acquire or to lose responses within a given learning paradigm then is widespread and not a measure which reliably differentiates between parts of the central nervous system or between animals with different kinds of nervous system. The ability to develop learning sets or strategies, that is to develop rules which speed the solution of problems, has at first sight a reasonable claim to be considered as a 'higher' form of adaptiveness than the ability to learn *per se*. The ability to form learning sets has received considerable attention as a possible differentiator between species and between different neural organizations (see also Chapter 6 of this volume).

Reversal learning sets

If a rat or a monkey is presented with a choice between two stimuli, for example two distinctively marked doors, and is always rewarded for choosing alternative A, it will slowly learn to make that choice and ignore alternative B. If the reward is then switched to alternative B, the animal makes more errors than it did during original learning but eventually comes to choose B in preference to A. If this reversal training procedure is repeated many times, however, the animal begins to reverse its choice rapidly, often only needing one trial to decide which is the rewarded door for that session. This improvement in performance marks the formation of a reversal learning set and, among a number of interpretations, may be seen as the progressive adoption of some form of win-stay, lose-shift strategy on the first one or two trials of every training session. Bitterman (1965) in a series of influential studies found that, whilst this effect seemed reliable in mammals, the two species of fish he tested,

African mouthbreeders and goldfish, showed no tendency to improve in speed of reversal learning up to 150 reversals. There were two interesting aspects to this result. First, it appeared to differentiate between different classes of vertebrates and, second, it differentiated an animal with no neocortex (fish) from one with neocortex (mammal). To take the second difference first, it might be predicted that removing neocortex from a mammal (rat, rabbit, etc.) would render it behaviourally, as well as anatomically, more like a fish. Bitterman in fact attempted this surgical reversal of evolution by removing some 70 per cent of neocortex from infant rats and testing them on serial reversal problems as adults. He found that the neodecorticated rats did indeed perform like fish and failed to show improvement over a series of visual (black-white) reversal problems, though with spatial (left-right) habit reversals they remained rat-like and showed progressive improvement in the rate of each reversal of the same problem.

As Bitterman's lesions were only 70 per cent removals of neocortex, it is possible that more complete lesions would render a mammal fish-like on spatial problems as well. Totally neodecorticated rabbits trained in a spatial discrimination in which they learned to press one of two identical treadles for food reward were given fifteen reversals of the same problem and showed no tendency to improve their rate of reversal learning when a sessions-to-criterion measure was used (Oakley, 1978). Taking the number of responses made to the incorrect treadle on the first day of each reversal, however, showed that the neodecorticates did learn to shift from the incorrect treadle sooner as training progressed (see Figure 7.2), though it is clear from the figure that the neodecorticates continued to make considerably more errors on the first day of each reversal than the normals at all stages of training. The failure to develop a visual reversal learning set after neocortical removal has been confirmed by Diamond and Hall (1969) in the tree shrew. The limited data so far available thus suggest that visual reversal learning is dependent on neocortex whilst spatial reversal learning sets are formed even in its absence, though the level of efficiency demonstrated so far in total neodecorticates is very low even after fifteen reversals on the same problem.

Whilst the view that reversal learning set formation is prevented or is at least impaired in mammals by neodecortication has not been seriously challenged, the phylogenetic distribution of learning set

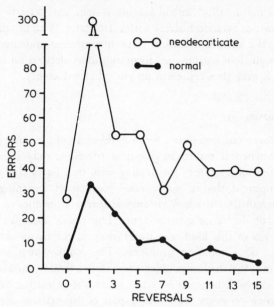

Fig. 7.2   Mean number of errors (responses to the incorrect treadle) on the first day of acquisition (Reversal 0) and the first day of subsequent reversals of a two treadle (left-right) discrimination for food reward in 6 normal and 2 neodecorticated rabbits. For clarity alternate reversals only are shown. Both groups of animals improved their performance after the first reversal on this measure.

ability has increasingly proved embarrassing to Bitterman's position. The fact that both birds and reptiles, neither of which have any significant development of neocortex, improve in both spatial and visual reversal learning series is difficult to accommodate, but more importantly subsequent studies using fish have demonstrated the formation of reversal learning sets on spatial as well as visual problems (see Warren, 1974). One species of fish, the Oscar, has proved particularly adept at forming reversal learning sets. Worse still, the humble woodlouse, an invertebrate crustacean, not only learns a spatial discrimination in a T-maze but forms a significant reversal learning set over just nine reversals (Morrow and Smithson, 1969). As with general learning ability it may be premature to identify this 'higher' ability to form learning sets too closely with any particular part of the mammalian central nervous system, with a particular type of vertebrate or even exclusively with vertebrates. With this disclaimer in mind, the neodecortication data nevertheless indicate that in mammals efficient learning set formation may depend on neocortex and that it may thus represent an encephalized ability.

General learning sets

The improvement seen over a series of reversals of the same problem, especially when it results in one-trial reversals, may indicate the development of a strategy for dealing with that particular problem, the development, that is, of a reversal learning set. Learning sets can also be demonstrated when an animal learns a number of different problems of the same general type. The classic demonstration of learning sets of this kind was by Harlow in rhesus monkeys using two-object discrimination problems. The monkey first learned to choose one of two dissimilar objects to obtain a food reward concealed in a shallow well beneath its base. Once the rewarded object was being chosen on every trial a new pair of objects was used as the discriminative stimuli and so on through a long series of different two-object discriminations. At first it took several choices before the monkey settled onto the consistently rewarded alternative but eventually they were able to solve each new problem in one trial. This particular form of learning-how-to-learn resulting in apparently insightful solution of new problems of a familiar type was for a number of years accepted as an index which would distinguish between animals on the basis of a conventional phylogenetic hierarchy and cortical complexity (see Warren, 1974). Gradually the neat picture in which rhesus monkey was better than squirrel monkey, squirrel monkey was better than cat, and cat better than rat became clouded. This was caused first of all by the huge variance which appeared between individual members of the same species – some cats were better than squirrel monkeys for instance. Of more importance, later studies using less conventional experimental subjects found that mink and ferrets formed learning sets at rates which were not unlike those of chimpanzees, reaching the 'insightful' one-trial solution stage. White Plymouth chickens perform on visual learning set problems as efficiently as cats and marmosets and apparently better than dolphins, whose intelligence and cortical complexity has otherwise been widely publicized. There is clearly little basis here for equating learning set performance with phylogenetic classification, degree of cortical development or, in view of the chicken data, the development of significant amounts of neocortex at all. The original rankings which put primates at the top of the mammalian learning set tree may have had more to do with the types of problem used than with neocortical complexity. The majority of learning set studies have employed colourful, three-dimensional 'junk' objects well suited to primate and, as it would now appear, to chicken, mink and ferret sensory capacities. It is tempting to agree with Warren (1974) that it might be possible to invert the monkey to rat learning set ranking if olfactory discriminations were used as the basis for a new series of learning set studies.

Neocortex and social interactions

Conventional learning designs of the sort employed in psychology laboratories then give rather few clues as to the unique selective advantages conferred by neocortex which might account for its emergence in the course of vertebrate evolution. The knack of solving evironmentally posed problems by learning had apparently been acquired by animals long before the evolution of neocortex. It is possible, however, that the adaptive significance of neocortex lies not with environmentally posed problems but with those posed by other animals, particularly those of the same species. The computing capacity required to handle social interactions with even a limited number of self-regulating individuals of the same species is likely on a number of grounds to be greater than that needed for interaction with the physical environment. The idea that social demands are a far more likely place to look for explanations of intellectual development than the simple technology of living has been forcefully argued by Humphrey (1976). Humphrey proposes as an illustration the literary observation of Defoe that Robinson Crusoe's problems in coming to terms with his environment were slight compared to the pressures created by the arrival of Man Friday. Add to this the possibility that Monday, Tuesday, Wednesday and Thursday, not to mention the female version of each, might turn up as well and the point becomes very clear. In fact Humphrey was concerned with why the usually conservative process of evolution should produce primates which were seemingly far too intelligent for their environments. Apes in the laboratory can display impressive feats of intellectual

achievement, ranging from one-trial solutions to object discriminations already mentioned and the use of tools and the building
of towers to reach food, described many years ago by Köhler, to
their recently described ability to communicate with their human
handlers by the use of sign language (Linden, 1976). Humphrey
compared such achievements with the lifestyle of the gorillas he
watched over a two-month period in the Virunga Mountains. They
lived by gathering the abundantly available food and did little
else but sleep and play. It is possible to assume that gorillas and
other apes have slipped back into a less demanding lifestyle
than that which initially favoured the massive development of
neocortex in primates. Alternatively we could take Humphrey's
point that, however simple the environment, the need for intellectual
power to handle social interactions, especially where the members of
the living chess game have moves which are predictable at best on
a statistical basis, remains. To generalize this point for the present
discussion we should have to assume that mammalian social
interactions have qualities different from those of other groups of
animals and that neocortex is a structure particularly suited to
carrying them out. We must also assume that mammalian social interactions contribute to evolutionary fitness.

From my own observations it is certainly true that rabbits and rats
without neocortex can handle their cage environments well. They
groom themselves, find food and water and generally look and behave
in ways which are very little different from other caged rabbits
and rats. The neodecorticated rabbits, along with the normals, have
even taken to rattling their cage-fronts as if to attract attention whenever an experimenter or technician enters the room around feeding
time. I do not know how they would handle a more natural environment and in particular how they would fare in social interactions
with other rabbits or rats. Clearly it is time to find out, especially
if we are to entertain seriously the notion of neocortex as a social
organ which has as its by-product high levels of function in apparently
non-social intellectual tasks.

I know of very few studies which relate social functions to neocortex.
Bignall and Schramm (1974) reared kittens which had been decerebrated within one week of birth and found that though a variety
of behavioural patterns such as auditory reflexes, placing reactions,
defensive and prey behaviour and thermoregulation appeared in
nearly normal chronological order this developmental process stopped

short of socialization. Some rather old studies by Beach are also perhaps relevant to the extent that sexual activity can be considered a 'social' behaviour (see Bermant and Davidson, 1974). Beach found that sexual activity in the male rat was abolished after neodecortication. The same is true of the male cat though not apparently of the male rabbit. Neodecortication does not, on the other hand, affect sexual responsiveness in female rats, rabbits, cats or dogs. Indeed removal of neocortical function by the application of potassium chloride to the brain surface seems to enhance the sexual responsiveness of female rats (Clemens et al., 1967). It is not entirely clear whether the deficit produced in males by loss of neocortex is one of motor control, of responsiveness to sensory cues or to some other factor entirely, though in the case of rats Beach concluded that it was the ease of arousal of sexual behaviour and not the ability to execute the behavioural patterns which was affected. It could be that the neodecorticated male fails to interpret the behavioural signals from the female appropriately. In our own studies we have found that neodecorticated male rats which had recently completed a series of tests during which they worked on an elevated chain manipulandum on an FR60 schedule for food in a very efficient manner were unwilling or unable to impregnate the receptive females we introduced to their home cages for a period of cohabitation. In view of the earlier equation of neocortex with 'higher' functions we have been led to wonder which represents the higher intellectual achievement for male rats – FR60 in a Skinner box or copulation with a female conspecific.

Neocortex and feeding

The unexpected involvement of neocortex with other, at first sight rather basic, activities has also emerged. We have consistently found that our neodecorticated rats and rabbits are lighter in weight than sham-operated control animals despite their apparent good health and a distinct tendency to eat more food than normals. The neodecorticates also respond more rapidly than normals to food deprivation, lose proportionately more weight over the same deprivation period and take longer to regain their pre-deprivation weights. All of this implies a higher metabolic rate in the absence of neocortex. In a similar vein Braun (1975) has reported that total neodecortication in rats results in finickiness (an abnormally strong tendency to be deterred by unpleasant tastes introduced into food or water), an increased tendency to drink whilst eating and a lower set-point for body weight. Again it is sobering when we search for higher functions mediated by neocortex to have also to consider body weight regulations as a process with a clear neocortical involvement.

Neocortex and sensory processes

Introduction

Perhaps we have indeed been too easily seduced by what is little more than an analogy between what we, perhaps egotistically, have considered a higher anatomical structure and the behaviours we expect to attribute to it. Neocortex after all evolved as a set of sensory analysers plus an area for motor control (Diamond and Hall, 1969). The neocortex of the most primitive mammals, represented perhaps by the modern hedgehog, and even those less primitive representatives, the rat and rabbit, is almost entirely taken up with visual, auditory, somatosensory and motor areas (see Chapter 2 of this volume). Even the proposition that neocortex evolved initially to serve sensory functions raises serious questions, however. The following will, for convenience, refer mainly to vision though the same principles apply to other cortical sensory areas as well as to motor cortex. The first and most fundamental problem is that it simply does not make good evolutionary sense to develop, at considerable cost in terms of space and energy requirements, an entirely new structure which in its early stages can do little more than replicate functions already carried out elsewhere in the central nervous system. The reptilian retina, midbrain and striatum serves as a perfectly adequate visual system which, moreover, can be elaborated without neocortex, as in birds, to provide visual functions to rival those of any mammal.

Cross-modal integration and matching

Why then encephalize vision by evolving costly neocortical structures – where is the competitive advantage? One possible advantage may lie in the fact that it is not just vision which has been neo-corticalized. The original olfactory forebrain functions have been joined on the surface of the hemisphere by neocortical sites for other major senses as well as vision. In the reptilian brain the auditory areas are rather differently located from those which subserve olfaction. The visual areas are at a distance from areas mainly responsive to touch and balance. In the mammalian brain, in addition to the old reptilian sensory sites, the senses are all gathered together in a single and comparatively homogeneous structure – the neocortex. This may be advantageous in facilitating the integration or cross-indexing of information from different sensory modalities about, say, an object of prey in the environment. It may in particular enable the animal to recognize a single aspect of its environment as being the same whether it is encountered as a visual stimulus, by touch or by smell. That is, to develop a polysensory image or model of significant objects or events. Any information which a predator, for example, gained on the basis of sight about its prey could then be attached to the feel, smell, sound etc. of that same object without a separate learning experience for each sensory modality.

Is there any evidence that animals can recognize objects as being the same even if they encounter them via different sensory modalities? Can they, in other words, carry out what has been labelled cross-modal matching (Weiskrantz, 1977)? A typical test for cross-modal matching is one in which the subject is allowed to feel, but not see, an object, such as a square wooden block, and is then presented with a selection of objects which he can see but not touch. The majority of human subjects are able to choose the square block from the visual sample, though performance is less good as the complexity of the objects increases. Adult humans might achieve this feat by linguistic means, by attaching the word 'square', in itself a variant of cross-modal matching, to the feel and then the sight of the object. Whilst linguistic mediation is clearly important it is not the sole mechanism of cross-modal matching as six-month-old children and chimpanzees have recently been shown to possess the ability. In the case of the chimpanzees the results were particularly impressive as the animals could perform touch to vision matching even if the visual representation of the solid objects was in the form of photographs, silhouettes or even line drawings. Weiskrantz and his associates developed an ingenious method of presenting essentially the same problem to rhesus monkeys and found similarly high levels of cross-modal matching ability. The monkeys were fed in total darkness with standard lab chow moulded into distinctive geometric shapes. Some of these shapes always tasted bad (they had sand and quinine mixed in) whilst the rest were unadulterated chow. When the monkeys were later allowed to choose shaped chow by vision alone they carefully avoided selecting shapes which had previously tasted unpleasant, indicating clear tactile to visual matching of shape. In line with a neocortical hypothesis for sensory integration this ability does seem to be impaired in monkeys following removal of areas of neocortex (see Weiskrantz, 1977). Whilst this is interesting from the point of view of primate neocortex it does not help greatly in understanding the evolution of neocortex unless the precursors of cross-modal matching can be found in other mammals with less well-developed neocortices.

Cross-modal transfer

I know of no studies showing cross-modal matching other than in primates but what appears at first sight to be a rather similar phenomenon, that of cross-modal transfer, has been shown in mouse, rat, rabbit and in a simple primate, the bushbaby (Ward et al., 1976). In a typical cross-modal transfer experiment the animal is trained to produce a response (commonly eyeblink or avoidance) to one frequency of light flashes (frequency A) but not to another frequency (B). Once the discrimination is well established, clicks at the same two frequencies are substituted for the light flashes. If the animal continues to respond to clicks at frequency A but not at frequency B, visual to auditory transfer of information seems to have taken place. Unfortunately there are problems in seeing this type of cross-modal ability as a simple version of cross-modal matching. In particular the animal could, and perhaps does, solve the problem by ignoring the sensory modality completely and attending simply to the on-off characteristics which are common to both sets of stimuli. Any elementary neural pool which was responsive to stimulation *per se* could presumably handle this problem without the need specifically to integrate distinct sensory information. Congruent with this is the fact that neocortical lesions which separate visual from auditory cortex do not impair cross-modal transfer from light to click stimuli in the bushbaby (Ward et al., 1976). This observation plus the rather broad distribution of cross-modal transfer across mammalian species suggested to Ward and his co-workers that this particular ability, even if it were in fact based on the integration of sensory information, may not depend on neocortex but on some 'phyletically old and conservative neural system'.

Simply separating two areas of neocortex, however, leaves rather a lot of neocortex intact, much of it polysensory in nature and I would feel much happier with Ward et al.'s conclusion if cross-modal transfer had been shown to survive total neodecortication. Moreover, some of our own earlier data encourages me to retain the neocortical sensory integration hypothesis at least until more convincing evidence is produced. We were training rabbits using a Pavlovian nictitating membrane conditioning procedure to discriminate between a 500 msec flash of light and a 500 msec duration tone and found to our surprise that totally neodecorticated animals were actually rather better at this discrimination than normals. They were less likely than normal animals to respond to the negative stimulus. This was particularly true under reversal conditions where the negative stimulus had previously served as the positive stimulus. Reversal was quicker and clearer in the neodecorticates. This puzzling 'improvement' caused by loss of neocortical tissue could even be demonstrated in animals which were trained as normals and then neodecorticated (see Figure 7.3). Tone-light discrimination was clearer after removal of neocortex than it had been before (Oakley and Russell, 1977).

Though admittedly *post hoc* and only one of several possible explanations the interpretation of these results which we suggested for future evaluation was that the normal animals were subjecting the sensory data to a higher level of integrative analysis which allowed them to generalize across the common features of both stimuli whereas the neodecorticates were treating each stimulus as a separate entity. The normals, in other words, might be using neocortex to compare light and tone and to recognize the common features of both (sudden onset, intense stimuli of 500 msec duration occurring in an otherwise constant environment). This integration would be expected to lead to a measurable tendency to treat both stimuli as equivalent and hence to respond to both, especially perhaps under response reversal conditions. The neodecorticates, on the other hand, could be seen as using their subcortical sensory sites to learn independently about light and tone. If light were always followed by shock and tone were not there would be no basis for the decorticate to respond to tone at all. Similarly, if the conditions were reversed so that tone was always followed by shock and light no longer was, the neodecorticates could learn to respond to tone and cease responding to light as two separate problems. The fact that removal of neocortex after normal learning

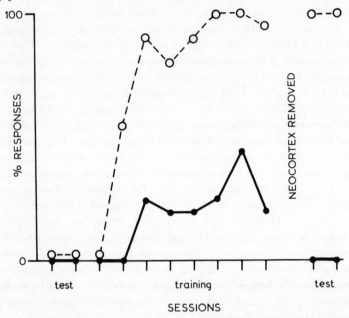

Fig. 7.3   A normal rabbit did not produce nictitating membrane (thrid eyelid) responses to either a light (dashed line) or a tone (solid line) when tested prior to Pavlovian conditioning (far left of figure). Pavlovian training, in which cheek shock always followed the light, established responses to that stimulus but also created a tendency to respond to the tone (middle section of the figure). Following surgical removal of all neocortex testing revealed that responses to light were retained but the animal had ceased responding to the tone (far right of figure). The retention of responses to light indicates subcortical storage of this information in the normal brain. The loss of responses to tone may be due to the removal of the integrating influence of neorcortex which led the animal to respond to features shared by two stimuli. The neodecorticate seems to treat these signals arriving via different sensory modalities as completely unrelated events.

did not abolish the discrimination implies that in the intact brain the subcortical sensory sites are normally used as a basis for Pavlovian discrimination with neocortical integration of sensory data as a separate and additional process. Removal of neocortex would improve discrimination performance by removing the integrating mechanism, and with it the tendency to respond to both stimuli, leaving the independent modality specific learning mediated by subcortex to control response emission.

Internal models

Related to the notion that neocortex serves to draw together sensory information for integration and comparison into a single structure is the already mentioned possibility that this would facilitate the building of effective polysensory models of the external world. The idea that brains can advance by creating internal models of their environments is commonly traced back to the writings of Craik (see Craik, 1943). This view accepts not only that the nature of reality depends on the brain which constructs it but it allows that reality to be symbolically manipulated. It allows the internal shuffling of objects and events (or at least their neuronal representations) and the prediction of possible outcomes which we categorize in human terms as reasoning or thinking. For example, if I wish to plan the construction of even so simple an object as a door frame I need to be able to represent in my brain the components, two uprights and a cross piece, and I also need central processes to represent the order in which I shall assemble the parts. I can try out in my mind placing the top piece first, one side piece and then the top or both side pieces then the top and in each case I can represent the consequences of that approach. Moreover, and herein lies a significant advantage, I can do so more rapidly than I could try out each approach in practice as well as avoiding damage to myself from falling timber – though I have a central representation of that possibility as well. It is also clear from this example that to be successful central models must be as accurate as possible especially when it comes to representing temporal order. Jerison (1973) points out that the recoding of a mass of sensory information as 'objects' in 'space' and 'time' may serve as subroutines which simplify the information processing task of the central nervous system. He also equates neural model building with consciousness and suggests that it did not reach significant levels until the evolution of mammals, though he concedes the possibility that it occurs in birds albeit to a lesser extent. Vertebrate species with less elaborate brains than mammals Jerison sees as transferring information from sensory to motor channels without the intervention of conscious modelling processes.

Encephalization of sensory functions

It is perhaps worth considering at this point what Craik's internal modelling view might mean in terms of encephalization of sensory functions and, again, visual function in particular. If neocortex evolved to provide new abilities, to provide a basis for integration across sensory modalities and to provide the raw material for the construction of manipulable models of the external world, there is no real need to assume that exisiting sensory abilities were encephalized. It may be useful in fact to retain a basic sensory system independently from the new modelling system in order to keep the latter free from direct sensory constraints. One of the traditional supports for the encephalization, and particularly the corticalization, of vision was that sensory loss after the removal of visual neocortex became progressively more severe as one 'ascended' a hypothetical phylogenetic hierarchy from rat to monkey, culminating in total blindness in man following striate neocortex damage (see Introduction and Chapter 2 and 6 of this volume and Weiskrantz, 1977).

More recent work, however, has shown that neither monkey nor man is completely blind without visual neocortex. Monkeys deprived of neocortex can apparently see patterns, develop three-dimensional spatial vision and conduct themselves quite ably in complex visual environments (Humphrey 1974). In man the picture is more complicated, but even more interesting, because there are basically two ways in which to assess visual function. One way is to take a patient who has sustained damage to his visual neocortex, present visual stimuli to his 'blind' visual field and ask him what he sees. If he reports seeing nothing we could take the information at its face value and conclude, as clinicians have done for decades, that damage to visual neocortex causes blindness. On the other hand, he could be tested in the way a monkey is tested by encouraging him to point to a screen whenever a stimulus of a particular sort appears on it. This is of course an odd thing for the patient to accept as a reasonable task as he is not aware of seeing anything at all on the screen. However, humans are co-operative creatures, even without the Smarties and raisins offered as inducements to other primates, and will perform the task if encouraged simply to 'guess' when a stimulus appears. One particular patient with damaged visual neocortex was able to point with remarkable accuracy to spots of light, to indicate whether lines were horizontal, vertical or diagonal and could discriminate between an O and an X. His visual acuity within the 'blind' visual field was normal when tested using line gratings. Nevertheless throughout all of these tests the patient continued to deny seeing anything at all and was openly surprised at the accuracy of his 'guesses' when his scores were revealed to him at the end of testing.

It appears then that the human patient without visual neocortex has an impressive array of visual functions – abilities which Weiskrantz and his co-workers have termed 'blindsight' (Weiskrantz, 1977). These data indicate that other areas of the brain, presumably the midbrain visual centres, are functional and that vision has not become encephalized even in man. What is even more striking though is that these residual visual functions remained outside consciousness and could not be acknowledged by the human subject. Simply asking a patient if he can see is clearly not the best way of establishing whether or not visual function is present; it is only a means of finding out whether he is consciously aware of that function. Similar problems arise when testing human amnesics – patients who appear to be unable to remember for more than a few minutes at a time. Weiskrantz and Warrington (1978) have shown, for instance, that even after several hundred eyeblink conditioning trials during which conditioned responses had been acquired and retained (i.e. remembered) over a twenty-four hour period, human amnesic patients still denied any memory of the conditioning procedure or of the apparatus.

The ability to solve visual pattern discriminations and to use spatial vision has also been shown in rat, tree shrew, rabbit, hedgehog, golden hamster and cat in the absence of visual neocortex, though it is not clear in all cases that the animals were using pure pattern perception rather than some other means, such as local brightness or flicker cues, as a basis for solution. Whether or not this implies visual control by other neocortical sites or by subcortical centres requires the careful testing of completely neodecorticate preparations. As yet we have only just begun to make this analysis, but the data obtained so far make it clear that totally neodecorticated rats are able to perform at high levels of efficiency on both acquisition and reversal of a horizontal-vertical stripe discrimination when tested in a straight alleyway for food reward.

Imagery

As there is little evidence for corticalization of sensory function in the mammalian brain, it seems reasonable to conclude at this stage that primitive subcortical sensory systems retain their full range of abilities.

On the basis of the human data it seems that neocortical sensory processing is associated with functions which enter consciousness and which are perhaps manipulable in the form of sensory images. In view of this we should perhaps accept for the time being Jerison's proposal that environmental modelling to any significant extent is not only a conscious process but also one which is predominantly the domain of mammals and in particular mammalian neocortex. Two examples may serve to indicate that animals do develop and utilize models of their environment and seem on occasion to base their behaviour on this model in preference to direct sensory information. Lorenz (1952) describes how water shrews once they have learned their way around their environment will continue to leap over an imaginary stone after the real stone has been removed from its accustomed place. Similarly Griffin (1976) recounts that bats in familiar surroundings will fly into newly placed objects or turn to avoid ones which have been removed even though their echolocation system is not only working but is quite able to distinguish the presence, or absence, of such objects. In more formal experiments conducted over a period of thirty years, Beritoff (Beritashvili, 1971) investigated what he called 'image-driven behaviour' in a range of vertebrates from fish to baboons and concluded that the use of imagery was exclusively a function of the forebrain and particularly of neocortex.

The basic paradigm which Beritoff adopted was to allow an animal to eat at a particular location in an unfamiliar room and then to reintroduce the animal hungry to the same room some time later. If the animal was able to go immediately to the location where it had previously fed, sometimes having to circumvent newly placed obstructions to do so, Beritoff concluded that this was evidence of a retained neural model or 'image' of the room and the relation of the feeding location to its major features. Using appropriate variations of this design he found that fish retained a usable image of the feeding location for only 8–10 seconds, reptiles (lizards) for 3–3$\frac{1}{2}$ minutes, birds (chickens) for 1–5 days, rabbits for 6–8 days, cat and dog for up to one month and the baboon for at least 1$\frac{1}{2}$ months. Consistent with this phylogenetic series which seems to equate degree of neocortical development very clearly with the durability of imagery, Beritoff found that total neodecortication in mammals abolished image-driven behaviour. The need for neocortical involvement for subjective 'image' formation is clearly in line with the human 'blindsight' data. The human patient without visual neocortex is evidently able to see but is not able to form conscious visual images.

Reasoning

Once central representations, models or images of environmental objects and events are formed they are potentially available for recombination in processes of 'thought' or reasoning. A direct approach to the question of reasoning ability in mammals was adopted by Maier. Maier devised a three-table reasoning task for rats in which the animal was first of all allowed to explore the three tables and three runways which linked them until it was completely familiar with the entire apparatus. (The tables typically had screens so that the animals could not see onto them from the runways.) This constituted Experience A, during which a polysensory mental image of the apparatus could be formed. The rat was then taken and placed on one of the tables and fed there. This was Experience B in which food was associated with a particular table. The rat was finally tested by being placed on one of the other two tables. The question was, could the rat combine the central representation of Experience B with that developed during Experience A and run directly to the table which previously held food. Could it, in other words, use a cognitive model or map of the three tables developed in Experience A as the basis for choosing the correct runway to get to the food table. Normal rats were successful on 80 per cent or more of test trials, but removal of as little as 22–4 per cent of neocortex, irrespective of locus, totally abolished 'reasoning' ability (for a typical experiment in this series see Maier, 1932). This result is interesting not only because it implicates neocortex in a behaviour which depends on the integration of central images but because of the small size of lesion required to abolish performance totally. Other studies in a similar vein carried out by Krechevsky at around the same time showed that equally small neocortical lesions in rats reduced the number of 'hypotheses' adopted in solving behavioural problems, reduced variability and increased stereotypy of behaviour and prevented the solution of Umweg (detour) problems (for a representative experiment in this series see Krechevsky, 1938). Behaviours which involve the development or utilization of environmental models or maps would thus appear to be particularly sensitive to neocortical damage, which is of course what a neocortical polysensory modelling hypothesis would predict.

Imagery and instrumental learning

In considering the role of neocortex in instrumental learning earlier in this chapter I concluded that neocortex was not needed for the successful demonstration of instrumental learning but that the course of acquisition was slower and the efficiency of performance in Skinner boxes was reduced in the neodecorticates unless specific pretraining was given. A neocortical modelling account may clarify this conclusion. I have spent many hours watching neodecorticated rabbits and rats working on treadle and bar manipulanda for food reward and have been impressed that whereas normals give the appearance of 'knowing' what they are doing the neodecorticates seem to perform the instrumental response without insight – sometimes even accidentally as part of a stereotyped response pattern they have acquired. It is customary for me to apologize quickly at this point for introducing subjective impressions into the argument in the guise of data. I have, however, tried to make some quantification of the behaviours giving rise to these impressions. If we assume first of all that normal animals develop a neocortical representation, or 'image' in Beritoff's sense, of the manipulandum as an object, they should continue to respond to it readily wherever it is placed in the environment. They might also perhaps be expected to transfer their pressing response from one object-to-be-manipulated to another. Normal rabbits do in fact seem able to follow a manipulandum as it is placed in different parts of the Skinner box and continue to operate it in the same manner. They will also readily shift their response from a treadle placed near the floor to a bar mounted higher on the wall. Neodecorticates have so far failed on both these tests of manipulandum identification. Extensive prior training aimed at drawing the animals' attention to the manipulandum and making it distinct from other aspects of the apparatus does seem to compensate the neodecorticates for their tissue loss (Oakley, 1978). Perhaps this could be seen as an instance of the experimenter substituting his own training procedures for the neocortex's normal ability to produce a polysensory model or cognitive map furnished with distinct and manipulable objects and relationships. Certainly the neodecorticate's inability to use a familiar manipulandum when it is moved to a new position in the apparatus suggests a rather rigid cognitive framework in which the rapid reorganization of elements is not possible. The neodecorticate, I am suggesting, can learn in the instrumental/associative sense that a particular stimulus or response is followed by a particular outcome but that it cannot form (conscious?) images with which to reason about its environment. This may not only make acquisition of instrumental responses less rapid, less 'insightful', but will render its behaviour less flexible in the face of rapid environmental change.

Social models

In relation to the earlier considerations of neocortex as a social organ it would follow that one of the most important sets of relationships which an animal might need to model would be that involving other individuals of its own species. Successful interactions within a group, especially a highly interdependent one as in social carnivores and primates, require an accurate central representation not only of the other members and their interrelations but also of likely reactions to the behaviour of the modeller himself. The modeller must therefore include a central representation of himself and the more accurate the self-model presumably the more successful will be the social interactions based on it. The advantages of central modelling of social interactions are similar to those of door-frame modelling. It is not only quicker but safer to try out social strategies by simulation using neural models than it is to risk direct confrontation, which an overt trial-and-error approach would entail. If neocortex were fashioned in a social mould and still bore that imprint it is perhaps not so surprising that the human mind has persistently sought to interact socially with its physical environment. God and the elements have been persuaded and placated; gardeners interact, sometimes verbally, with their charges in a proto-social fashion and we still find a strange fascination in the idea that cutlery may be bent just by wishing it (see Humphrey, 1976).

Neocortex and consciousness

The fundamental problem in considering the relation of consciousness to any particular neurological structure or assembly of neurones is that of defining consciousness itself. As individuals we experience a subjective state which we label as consciousness and we believe, but can presumably never directly know, that a similar state is present in those around us. Perhaps, as Ornstein (1972) suggests, the quest for a textbook definition is futile and the only way to define consciousness is to experience it. Griffin (1976), on the other hand, offers a working definition of consciousness as the presence of mental images and their use by an animal to regulate its behaviour. Part of the problem is also that consciousness is a blanket-term covering a number of quantitatively and perhaps qualitatively different states.

At possibly its simplest level consciousness implies an ability to respond to external events. We may readily accept that a rat responding to a light is in some sense conscious of that particular stimulus, but does the celandine as it opens its petals at daybreak share this awareness of the stimuli acting upon it, and what about a photographic plate? Somewhere along the line we have made a value judgement if we agree that the photographic plate was not conscious of the light to which it reacted. Perhaps we would like to limit consciousness to living systems, to animals even and in particular to their nervous systems. To do so we must choose to ignore the strong similarities which exist between 'neural' conduction pathways in plants and animals (Sanberg, 1976). If consciousness depends on neurones and their activity, as I assume it must, and as all neurones, invertebrate or vertebrate, reptilian or mammal, are remarkably similar there is no *a priori* reason for denying consciousness to any one collection of neurones and allowing it in another (Doty, 1975).

This physiologically based argument for the continuity of consciousness is paralleled by the evolutionary one. If we accept that the human brain, where we know consciousness to exist, evolved through a continuous and gradual process of change, the most parsimonious view must be that consciousness also evolved in the same way and that differences in consciousness between man and the rest of the animal kingdom, especially between man and the rest of the primates, are quantitative rather than qualitative (Griffin, 1976; Jerison, 1973). Provided we recognize that what we are doing in making more specific definitions of consciousness is to some extent arbitrary we can, however, profitably proceed a little further.

The ability of any information processing system to gather enough data about the outside world to create an internal model with which to simulate external events has been seen by many as an advance worthy of special consideration and perhaps a specific label. As indicated earlier Griffin (1976) and Jerison (1973) among others seem prepared to equate consciousness with internal modelling of the environment, the creation that is of manipulable 'images'. Jerison further equated this activity primarily with neocortex and, working in an entirely different framework, Beritoff (1971) concluded that 'imagery' was a product of neocortical tissue. The work of Weiskrantz (1977), cited earlier, also indicates that for visual information to be consciously available in human subjects it must be processed through neocortical tissue. If we are to limit arbitrarily consciousness to neural systems which form environmental models, use images and reason, the data reviewed in this chapter would lead us to equate consciousness with neocortex. Animals without neocortex might then be said to show 'awareness' but not consciousness. It must be admitted, however, that the neatness of this scheme is achieved by ignoring birds. Avian evolution from reptilian stock parallels that of mammals and both Beritoff and Jerison recognize that some exceptions from their generalizations must be allowed to accommodate birds. If consciousness is defined as the use of environmental models and 'images', Beritoff's data indicate consciousness in birds. They have, however, developed forebrain structures other than neocortex as the hardware for achieving this end. It must also be recognized that, as there are degrees of neocortical development in vertebrates generally and mammals in particular, consciousness must also be a graded entity.

In fact it seems necessary to adopt a special category of 'consciousness' to incorporate the very exciting data obtained from human split-brain subjects (see Chapters 8 and 9 of this volume). When the cerebral hemispheres of a human subject are surgically separated the patient regards himself as his left (speech) hemisphere. He is unaware of any of the imagery and complex cognitive activities taking place in his right hemisphere. When he is asked a question his left hemisphere answers. Moreover, he does not feel post-operatively that half his mind is missing or that his awareness has been reduced. In a similar manner to the amnesic patients and those with visual neocortex damage, the split-brain human denies what, to an observer, is clearly present: in this case the existence of 'consciousness' in his own right hemisphere. The special category of consciousness which these data seem to demand may be labelled perhaps as 'awareness of consciousness' or, less clumsily, as self-awareness, the basis of personal identity. It is compelling, though possibly mistaken, to identify self-awareness not only with neocortex but with a particular area of neocortex in one hemisphere – Wernicke's speech area. Perhaps this type of consciousness was the one we had in mind all along. If so, its existence raises a number of as yet unanswered questions: Is it purely human? Is it linked exclusively to language? Do chimps like Washoe now have self-awareness along with their new-found linguistic ability? Is it possible that all animals have self-awareness? Would a human reared without the use of language lack self-awareness? As with the two hemispheres of the human split-brain patient the most direct way to find out if self-awareness is present is to ask the individual concerned. Even so if Washoe or one of a new generation of computers answered 'Yes', would we believe them? The question of awareness in animals and proposals for a new science of cognitive ethology based on two-way communication between ethologists and animals are presented in a small, provocative volume by Griffin (1976).

Summary and conclusions

The idea that neocortex evolved to subserve learning or that it has progressively taken over that role in mammals, despite its initial attractiveness as an hypothesis, has little to support it, though there is some evidence that learning set formation may be an encephalized function in mammals. A more promising approach at the moment seems to be to consider that neocortex evolved because it provided a basis for the integration of sensory processes and ultimately for the formation of polysensory representations or models of the animals world. The manipulation of these central respresentations, or 'images', represents reasoning and thinking. I have spent rather little time on the later evolution of neocortex, especially human neocortex. I hope this is a justifiable bias when taking an evolutionary perspective. Apart from being nonsensical in terms of evolutionary theory, it would plainly be arrogant to consider that neocortex evolved to provide humans with language for instance. On the other hand, I believe that the major aspects of human cerebral specialization can be seen as derivatives of the more general processes which have been attributed to neocortex in this chapter. Language, in most people a left hemisphere process, has long been considered as a special case of sensory integration and cross-modal matching. Language also requires a modelling system which can preserve the strict temporal order of events, sounds in this case, and preserve them as patterns over time. There is good evidence that neocortex is specialized for this ability (Diamond and Neff, 1957; Weiskrantz, 1977). Furthermore, the pre-linguistic ability to utilize auditory imagery to solve behavioural problems appears to be a function of a small area of left hemisphere neocortex in the rhesus monkey (Dewson, 1977). Linguistic representations additionally form the basis for much internal modelling and particularly the manipulation of internal representations and re-presentations not only of physical objects and relationships but of abstractions deriving from them. The spatial/constructional abilities of the right hemisphere can perhaps be seen in terms of elaborate environmental mapping or modelling. An excellent introduction to human neuropsychology which expands these points can be found in Luria (1973).

The adaptive significance of effective environmental modelling by neocortex in guiding learning and behaviour generally has, I hope, emerged as the chapter progressed. If consciousness and self-awareness are seen simply as correlates of this modelling process there is no need to suggest a further adaptive significance for their subjective aspects. Any data processing system, animal or otherwise, which develops and manipulates environmental models, including self-models, and perhaps also monitors the modelling process itself may share the experience of consciousness. Alternatively, consciousness and self-awareness may represent the operation of some as yet unsuspected process which transcends information processing. Whatever this process might be the logic of evolutionary theory would lead us to assign some adaptive advantage to it.

Note

1   I would like to thank Professor L. Weiskrantz for his comments on an earlier version of this chapter.

References

Bard, P. and Mountcastle, V. B. (1948) Some forebrain mechanisms involved in expression of rage with special reference to suppression of angry behavior. *Research Publications of the Association in Nervous and Mental Disease 27*: 362–404.

Beritashvili, I. S. (J. S. Beritoff) (1971) *Vertebrate Memory: Characteristics and Origin*. New York: Plenum Press.

Berlucchi, G. and Buchtel, H. A. (1975) Some trends in the neurological study of learning. In M. S. Gazzaniga and C. Blakemore (eds) *Handbook of Psychobiology* London: Academic Press, 481–98.

Bermant, G. and Davidson, J. M. (1974) *Biological Basis of Sexual Behavior.* New York: Harper and Row.

Bignall, K. E. and Schramm, L. (1974) Behaviour of chronically decerebrated kittens. *Experimental Neurology 42*: 519–31.

Bitterman, M. E. (1965) Phyletic differences in learning. *American Psychologist 20*: 396–410.

Bjursten, L.-M., Norrsell, K. and Norrsell, U. (1976) Behavioural repertory of cats without cerebral cortex from infancy. *Experimental Brain Research 25*: 115–30.

Braun, J. J. (1975) Neocortex and feeding behavior in the rat. *Journal of Comparative and Physiological Psychology 89*: 507–22.

Bromiley, R. B. (1948) Conditioned responses in a dog after removal of neocortex. *Journal of Comparative and Physiological Psychology 41:* 102–10.

Buchwald, J. S. and Brown, K. A. (1973) Subcortical mechanisms of behavioral plasticity. In J. D. Maser (ed.) *Efferent Organization and the Integration of Behavior.* London: Academic Press, 99–136.

Chopin, S. F. and Buerger, A. A. (1975) Graded acquisition of an instrumental avoidance response by the spinal rat. *Physiology and Behaviour 15*: 155–8.

Clemens, L. G., Wallen, K. and Gorski, R. A. (1967) Mating behavior: facilitation in the female rat after cortical application of potassium chloride. *Science 157*: 1208–9.

Craik, K, J. W. (1943) *The Nature of Explanation* London: Cambridge University Press.

Dewson, J. H. (1977) Preliminary evidence of hemispheric asymmetry of auditory function in monkeys. In S. Harnad, R. W. Doty, L. Goldstein, J. Jaynes and G. Krauthamer (eds) *Lateralization in the Nervous System.* New York: Academic Press, 63–71.

Diamond, I. T. and Hall, W. C. (1969) Evolution of neocortex. *Science 164*: 251–62.

Diamond, I. T. and Neff, W. D. (1957) Ablation of temporal cortex and discrimination of auditory patterns. *Journal of Neurophysiology 20*: 300–15.

DiCara, L. V., Braun, J. J. and Pappas, B. A. (1970) Classical conditioning and instrumental learning of cardiac and gastrointestinal responses following removal of neocortex in the rat. *Journal of Comparative and Physiological Psychology 73*: 208–16.

Doty, R. W. (1975) Consciousness from neurons. *Acta Neurobiologiae Experimentalis (Warsaw) 35*: 791–804.

Girden, E., Mettler, F. A., Finch, G. and Culler, E. (1936) Conditioned responses in a decorticate dog to acoustic, thermal and tactile stimulation. *Journal of Comparative Psychology 21*: 367–85.

Griffin, D. R. (1976) *The Question of Animal Awareness: Evolutionary Continuity of Mental Experience.* New York: Rockefeller University Press.

Humphrey, N. K. (1974) Vision in a monkey without striate cortex: a case study. *Perception 3*: 241–55.

Humphrey, N. K. (1976) The social function of intellect. In P. P. G. Bateson and R. A. Hinde (eds) *Growing Points in Ethology*. Cambridge: Cambridge University Press, 303–17.

Huston, J. P. and Borbély, A. A. (1974) The thalamic rat: general behavior, operant learning with rewards hypothalamic stimulation and effects of amphetamine. *Physiology and Behavior 12*: 433–48.

Jerison, H. J. (1973) *Evolution of the Brain and Intelligence*. New York: Academic Press.

Krechevsky, I. (1938) Brain mechanisms and umweg behavior. *Journal of Comparative Psychology 25*: 147–73.

Lashley, K. S. (1929) *Brain Mechanisms and Intelligence*. Chigaco: University Press.

Light, A. R. and Durkovic, R. G. (1977) US intensity and blood-pressure effects on classical conditioning and sensitization in spinal cat. *Physiological Psychology 5*: 81–8.

Linden, E. (1976) *Apes, Men and Language*. New York: Penguin.

Lorenz, K. (1952) *King Solomon's Ring*. London: Methuen.

Luria, A. R. (1973) *The Working Brain: An Introduction to Neuropsychology*. Harmondsworth: Penguin.

Mackintosh, N. J. (1974) *The Psychology of Animal Learning*. London: Academic Press.

Maier, N. R. F. (1932) Cortical destruction of the posterior part of the brain and its effect on reasoning in rats. *Journal of Comparative Neurology 56*: 179–214.

McConnell, J. V. and Jacobson, A. L. (1974) Learning in invertebrates. In D. A. Dewsbury and D. A. Rethlingshafer (eds) *Comparative Psychology: A Modern Survey*. Tokyo: McGraw-Hill Kogakusha, 429–70.

Morrow, J. E. and Smithson, B. L. (1969) Learning sets in an invertebrate. *Science 164*: 850–1.

Norman, R. J., Buchwald, J. S. and Villablanca, J. R. (1977) Classical conditioning with auditory discrimination of the eye blink in decerebrate cats. *Science 196:* 551–3.

Oakley, D. A. (1971) Instrumental learning in neodecorticate rabbits. *Nature (New Biology) 233*: 185–7.

Oakley, D. A. (1978) Instrumental reversal learning and subsequent Fixed Ratio performance on simple and GO-NOGO schedules in neodecorticate rabbits. *Physiological Psychology*.

Oakley, D. A. and Russell, I. S. (1977) Subcortical storage of Pavlovian conditioning in the rabbit. *Physiology and Behavior 18*: 931–7.

Oakley, D. A. and Russell, I. S. (1978) Performance of neodecorticated rabbits in a free-operant situation. *Physiology and Behaviour 20*: 157–70.

Ornstein, R. E. (1972) *The Psychology of Consciousness*. San Francisco: W. H. Freeman.

Pavlov, I. P. (1927) *Conditioned Reflexes: An Investigation of the Physiological Activity of the Cerebral Cortex* (translated by G. V. Anrep). London: Oxford University Press.

Plotkin, H. C. and Odling-Smee, F. J. (in press) Learning, change and evolution: an enquiry into the teleonomy of learning. *Advances in the Study of Behaviour 10*.

Russell, I. S. (1966) Animal learning and memory. In D. Richter (ed.) *Aspects of Learning and Memory*. London: Heinemann, 121–71.

Sanberg, P. R. (1976) 'Neural capacity' in *Mimosa pudica*: a review. *Behavioral Biology 17*: 435–52.

Schwartz, B. and Gamzu, E. (1977) Pavlovian control of operant behavior: analysis of autoshaping and its implications for operant conditioning. In W. K. Honig and J. E. R. Staddon (eds) *Handbook of Operant Behavior*. Englewood Cliffs, New Jersey: Prentice-Hall, 53–97.

Stettner, L. J. and Matyniak, K. A. (1968) The brain of birds. *Scientific American 218* (6): 64–76.

Tighe, T. J. and Leaton, R. N. (1976) *Habituation: Perspectives from Child Development, Animal Behavior and Neurophysiology*. Hillsdale, New Jersey: Lawrence Erlbaum Associates.

Ward, J. P., Silver, B. V. and Frank, J. (1976) Preservation of cross-modal transfer of a rate discrimination in the bushbaby (*Galago senegalensis*) with lesions of posterior neocortex. *Journal of Comparative and Physiological Psychology 90*: 520–7.

Warren, J. M. (1974) Learning in vertebrates. In D. A. Dewsbury and D. A. Rethlingshafer (eds) *Comparative Psychology: A Modern Survey*. Tokyo: McGraw-Hill Kogakusha, 471–509.

Weiskrantz, L. (1977) Trying to bridge some neuropsychological gaps between monkey and man. *British Journal of Psychology 68*: 431–45.

Weiskrantz, L. and Warrington, E. K. (in press) Conditioning in amnesic patients. *Neuropsychologia*.

8 Symmetry and asymmetry in the vertebrate brain[1]

Stuart J. Dimond

Introduction

Michael Tippett the composer reminds us of the problem of duality
and yet unity in man when he says, talking of his piano sonatas, 'I
do get very fascinated with the hands as two distinct objects and
yet it is one human being playing'. When we approach the problems
of the brain the question of the coexistence of a fundamental
duality as well as a fundamental unity is raised even more vividly.
How is it that the brain exists as a double structure and yet is
still capable of producing the unified thread of conscious mental
experience?

Among the first expressions of the concept of the duality of the mind
was one published in 1844 by Wigan who observed that:

> Each cerebrum is a distinct and perfect whole.... A separate and
> distinct process of thinking ... may be carried on in each
> cerebrum simultaneously.... In the healthy brain one of the cerebra
> is almost always superior in power to the other, and capable of
> exercising control over the volitions of its fellow, and of preventing
> them from passing into acts or from being manifested to others.
> (Wigan, 1844, p. 26)

A number of other authors subsequently took up this theme. Hughlings Jackson in 1874, for example, published an article called 'On the nature of the duality of the brain'. From his clinical observations he concluded that the left half of the brain is that by which we speak; the right is the half by which we receive propositions. He came to the conclusion that for most people the left side of the brain is the leading side, the side of the so-called will, and that the right is the automatic side. Brown-Sequard (1874) also took up the question of the dual character of the brain. He held that we have two brains perfectly distinct the one from the other. If we make use of only one for most of our actions we leave useless one half of the most important of our organs as regards manifestations of intelligence, will and perception or sensation.

Whilst the duality of the brain remained important in some quarters, particularly with respect to the problems of language organization and cerebral dominance, in other quarters these ideas of duality were accorded only token recognition. The tradition grew to talk of the brain as singular both as an object in itself and with regard to the regions it contains (e.g. the temporal lobe) without in fact making a distinction between the two sides whatever the difference in their function. I believe that this tendency to regard the brain as a unitary thing was the result of a deep rooted conviction that, as experience is unitary, the system upon which experience depends must also be a simple complete unit. This inextinguishable view held by man about himself and born out of individual experience, was the factor I believe which resulted in the lack of acceptance of the ideas of the early pioneer neurologists as they concerned not only the duality of the brain but also disconnection of the elements of the person. An account of early views on brain asymmetry is given in Oppenheimer (1977).

In 1962, however, the picture radically changed. Young (1962) asked 'Why do we have two brains?' and argued that one important reason was the need for bilateral mapping of space associated primarily with binocular vision. He argued that a double brain is better than a single brain to map and preserve the essential isomorphic spatial relationships of the world. Secondly, Geschwind and Kaplan (1962) reported a case of cerebral disconnection in which damage to the splenium of the corpus callosum and visual cortex separated the hemispheres and destroyed the vision of the left hemisphere. The patient could see with the right hemisphere but could not describe what had been seen because the left (speaking) hemisphere was disconnected from the right (seeing) hemisphere. Inherent in the study of this case was the notion that parallel strands of mental action run in a separate flow in the two hemispheres. The third critical event occurring in 1962 was the publication of the case report on the first split-brain patient of the modern Californian series (Bogen and Vogel, 1962) so brilliantly examined and reported subsequently by Sperry, Gazzaniga and others. The human split-brain operation was used to control epilepsy and consisted of cutting the corpus callosum and other large fibre tracts which normally interconnect the cerebral hemispheres (see also Chapters 2 and 9 of this volume). Sperry (1964) showed that the split-brain symptoms reported previously for animals were also present for man and provided a powerful demonstration of the possibility of the existence of an independent mental life in each disconnected hemisphere (Gazzaniga, 1967; Sperry, 1968). It was, I submit, the dramatic demonstration of the mental pluralism of split-brain man (disputed even now by some) which presented a major challenge to the idea of the indestructible unity of human experience and which led to the current tide of interest in the question of the two halves of the brain and what they do. The question of laterality, symmetry and other features related to laterality have now been reinstated as of fundamental importance to modern neuroscience.

Patterns of symmetry and asymmetry in the vertebrate brain

Some emphasis has already been given to the historical concept of the duality of the brain. It remains, however, as one of the outstanding facts of the architecture of the brain that there exists a remarkable symmetry between one side and the other. The most obvious parts of the brain to external inspection to show this doubleness are the cerebral hemispheres but subcortical structures (hippocampi, thalami, amygdalae, etc), including those of the brainstem, are for the most part also paired. This feature of the brain arose extremely early in evolution and as a distinguishing mark it is to be found in invertebrates as well as in vertebrates. It is my belief that during the major transition from invertebrate forms the emerging vertebrates brought with them a nervous system in which bilateral symmetry was already a major feature. The dual nervous system, in other words, distinguishes modern and ancient forms alike, and I find it impossible to believe that the first vertebrate had only a straight tube of a nervous system, undifferentiated in any of its lateral parts, as many would have us believe.

Observations made on the first known primitive fish show that the brain was divided into the five typical regions and that the lateral structures were much as we recognize them today. The first known vertebrate, therefore, possessed a brain essentially similar in basic plan to that of vertebrates today, and the bilateral nervous system was as much a feature then as now (see Chapter 2 of this volume). There are, however, exceptions to this general rule of symmetry and perhaps these exceptions by virtue of contrast speak more eloquently to the point about symmetry than anything else we could say. Let us look therefore not at the symmetry but at asymmetry to observe the lessons this teaches us about the construction of the brain.

It was commonly thought that animal species other than man did not show asymmetry of brain function but recent work shows this generalization to have been quite mistaken. It may be said that the brain structure of fishes is as far removed from man as is possible within the vertebrates and if asymmetry was a unique feature of the brain of man then it should distinguish the brain of fish least of all. It is surprising, therefore, that asymmetries of structure in the fish brain not only exist but were present at least as long ago as the Devonian era. Preparations of some of the early fish skulls, for example, indicate unequal brain development because the parietal apertures do not match on the two sides. Brain asymmetries are also reported for many living fish forms, particularly around the roof region of the diencephalon. The reason for these asymmetries of fish brain and their functional significance remains completely unknown as does the reason for some of the other asymmetries which we shall now discuss.

The habenular nuclei are a focus for asymmetry in the amphibian brain as well as the fish brain. In one study of fifty frog brains all without exception showed a striking asymmetry of this structure. Other examples of asymmetry are reported by Nottebohm (1977) for some song bird species. In a recent review of this work he describes how section of the nerve leading through to the Syrinx (vocal organ) from the left side results in the almost total abolition of the song, but if the nerve is cut on the other side the song remains virtually unaltered. This remarkable demonstration of left-sided control of song is immediately reminiscent of man with his left hemisphere having responsibility for speech in most individuals. Nottebohm has tracked down the particular area of the brain involved. Lesions at the left side in an area of hyperstriatum cause a great disturbance in the production of song. This region is in addition anatomically different from the region on the opposite side and the two can be distinguished by their structure. The situation is still under investigation, however, and whilst lateralization and cerebral dominance has been found for canaries, chaffinches and song sparrows, other birds such as, the Amazonian parrot and the domestic hen do not show it at all. The lateralization of song in birds therefore remains as yet one more mystery revealed by modern research on the asymmetry of the brain.

The idea that some asymmetries may be correlated with brain biochemistry (see Chapter 4 of this volume) is an important one for further exploration. For some species the asymmetries do not distinguish each member of the species equally, neither are they all found to follow the same direction. Handedness in the laboratory rat, for example, is a marked feature of some animals but not others, and the number of animals exhibiting left preference roughly equals those showing right preference. Research on this topic shows that preference for right or left body turning is activated largely by the different dopamine levels in the two sides of the brain. Yet another important and largely unexplored aspect of the brain concerns the fissure patterns of the cerebral hemispheres. These can be classified into four or five different types in the cat, and in approximately half of the cat brains studied the fissure patterns were different on the two sides of the brain. The exact functional significance of these fissure patterns remains to be established.

Monkeys do not show the handedness patterns of man nor had their brains been found to show asymmetries of structure and it was generally concluded that the asymmetries so typical of the brain of man were not present in monkeys. Recently, however, this conclusion has been cast in doubt by the work of Dewson et al. (1975). These workers found that after destruction of part of the superior temporal gyrus (an area of the temporal lobe roughly corresponding to the classical Wernicke speech area in man) on the left side, monkeys were unable to carry out auditory matching tasks which involved a delay. These effects were not observed for damage to the corresponding contralateral area and controls were performed to make sure that the receiving part of the auditory brain at the cortex was not responsible.

Thus from an almost totally negative picture we move to one which depicts a widespread incidence of lateralization. Evidence has also accumulated latterly of an anatomical disparity between the two hemispheres for the higher apes and man. Once again the Sylvian fissure is involved, the region associated with the speech process in man. The gorilla, chimpanzee and the orangutan all show asymmetry of the brain in this region and in the majority of animals the asymmetry favours the left side. This striking modern evidence is causing a revision of thinking about the nature of brain asymmetry. We are now led to view the asymmetry of the human brain not as the unique distinguishing mark of man but as part of an historical development embracing other species.

It remains now to consider the human brain and to assess the contribution which asymmetries have made to its evolution. Clear anatomical asymmetries have been reported recently for the human brain involving the Sylvian fissure and planum temporale, which as we have already noted are areas of major importance to speech (Geschwind, 1972). In the Chapelle aux Saints skull of Neanderthal man dating back some 30,000 years the imprint of the Sylvian fissures is visible on both sides. That on the right side is angled up more sharply indicating that asymmetry was already present early in man's history. Studies of the brain of modern man conducted over the last ninety years consistently demonstrate the asymmetry within the region of the planum temporale. Many of the early studies pointed out the variations from one brain to another suggesting that although the asymmetry is most usually present it is so on a rather idiosyncratic basis. Similarly, in a more modern study of 100 normal adult brains the posterior margin of the Sylvian fissure was angled backward more sharply on the left in 57 per cent of the cases, on the right in 18 per cent of cases and approximately equal in 25 per cent of the cases. From the time of the earliest observations it has also been noted that the asymmetries are present in the brains of foetuses and the newborn. They therefore precede early environmental experience and it is extremely unlikely, therefore, that they occur as a result of experience. These are not the only asymmetries reported however. The pyramidal tracts, the largest of the descending motor systems, cross over first in the vast majority of cases from the left hemisphere, thereby suggesting differential rates of growth for the two hemispheres (Corballis and Morgan, 1978). The systems of ventricles of the brain also differ at the two sides. The left occipital horn is typically larger than the one on the right. Differences in the pattern of blood flow as well as the distribution of veins are similarly reported for the two hemispheres.

The conclusion must be, therefore, that anatomical diffrerences of a measurable kind exist between one half of the human brain and the other, and that the evolutionary picture is one of far greater continuity between mankind and other species in this respect than we may have thought possible until just a few years ago. The question of the significance of asymmetry, whether this be of anatomy or of function, is something that still remains to be discussed. For a fuller review of brain asymmetry see Dimond and Blizard (1977) and Harnad et al. (1977).

Evolutionary significance of bilaterality and the lateralization of the brain

I have emphasized doubleness as a feature of the brain and pointed out that a striking feature is its division into two halves. The question which confronts us now is: What is the reason for the brain to exist as a bilateral organ? It is clear that we have to search for the answer far back in evolutionary time because the vertebrates at their very inception already represented a stage of bilateral development. If we think of the organism as moving head first and transferring food into its centrally placed mouth then much of the bilateral symmetry of its organization will follow as a consequence of this. Gravity will act on the organism to keep it flat on the surface and the natural tendency would be for the organs to spread bilaterally around the fixed position of the centrally placed mouth and gut. In this respect the brain reflects other aspects of body symmetry and does not necessarily stand apart from these. One may assume that the possession of a bilateral brain conferred many advantages on its possessor and that it therefore remained preserved as a feature to distinguish the brains of all advanced species.

One of the most important functions of the brain is the creation of maps of the world. These should not be thought of merely as static pictures but rather a continuously changing up-dated registration of what takes place in the world around the organism. The highly encephalized brain cannot rest content with a flat two-dimensional sensory picture painted upon the retina or other senses. There must be a constructed three-dimensional inner world which mirrors depth and distance in the external environment. One model for the construction of a three-dimensional picture from an original two-dimensional source is that used to obtain information about distant stars and nebulae in the universe from a position here on earth. Two tracking stations from widely separated locations track the same object in space. In large measure the information obtained from each source is the same but there are also subtle differences. When the information from the two sources is combined then similarities and differences allow the recreation of the picture in all its three dimensional quality. The brain I believe is not vastly different from this. The world is scanned from different lateral sense organs, the information goes for analysis to different halves of the brain. Each half brain views the world from a slightly different position. It is the mutual exchange of derived information which allows the brain to reconstruct its three-dimensional picture of the world, but more importantly to operate in its three-dimensional structure and to use this 'sixth sense' in its fight for survival. The lateral brains can therefore be seen as providing an advanced system of information which goes beyond the surface information reaching the senses. I believe that this was a crucial step in the evolution of higher mental function.

The question of three-dimensional construction in perception is not the only one that can be addressed through consideration of the brain as a bilateral system. If two people are walking along a road and one is in danger of slipping on a banana skin then the other will certainly point this out to him. Together they form a team more vigilant than the person alone. On many occasions, particularly those concerned with survival, two are better than one, and in this particular circumstance the engagement of what amounts to two independent systems for perceptual analysis has an immense value to be placed upon it.

One of the most important reasons why evolution should have fashioned a bilateral brain and used it to such good purpose is that it can be seen even in its most primitive form as a system for guiding the organism towards certain target stimuli, particularly food and other resources, and equally away from sources of danger and threats to existence. Something of this can be seen in tropistic behaviour when the animal is unable to escape the bilateral urges of its brain. The moth propelled towards the light is a case in point. The animal is enmeshed in its motor activity which guides it forwards on a course of self-destruction. Some remnant of this may well exist in the bilateral arrangement of reflex systems for balance and co-ordinated bilateral activity.

The bilateral brain mechanisms of the motor system are of interest not only because they provide a highly integrated system by which the organism can focus the thrust of its activity in one central direction but also because in other circumstances the limbs can be disengaged from this co-ordinated pattern and act as independent machines on their own account. The female ape can feed with one hand, for example, whilst she clutches her infant at the same time with the other. Nature sometimes faces the organism with an environment in which the independence of lime function may be as important to survival as the totally co-ordinated pattern.

The idea that the bilaterality of the brain extends to functions other than simple sensory or motor abilities is an important one at the present time. In particular it may provide for greater diversity of mental activity. Bogen (1971) for instance stated 'The evolutionary advantage of having two different minds is obvious: possession of two independent problem-solving organs increases mightily the likelihood of a creative solution to a novel problem.' Witelson (1977) pointed out that it would be a waste of storage space to have duplication of functions in both hemispheres and Levy (1977) believes that for man certainly, and for the more highly differentiated mammals possibly, the allocation of separate cognitive functions to the two sides of the brain and the doubling of the effective size of the cognitive computer is invaluable. The relationship between brain asymmetry and the evolution of intelligence, advanced mental qualities and cognitions is considered further in Dimond (1978).

A related question concerning the design of the nervous system is that of crossed lateral control. One strange feature of the brain is that systems of control and the major sensory systems have rotated upon the central axis so that mechanisms on the left side come to control functions of the right side and vice versa. What happens in effect is that the main sensory receiving areas for the right side of the body are now located at the left hemisphere of the brain and vice-versa. Likewise for the systems of motor control. The main control systems for the right side of the body are located on the left side of the brain and vice-versa. The exact reason for this arrangement remains something of a mystery.

The next problem concerns asymmetry and the respective power which this gives to brain arrangements. It has already been argued that asymmetry is a more pervasive feature of evolutionary history than has generally been recognized. It is particularly the case here that general problems of brain organization cannot be considered totally in isolation from the development of other body systems which may have a bearing on them. The formation of a bilateral nervous system may have resulted from allocation of space around other central structures (e.g. the mouth and gut) and where asymmetries of brain are found it may well be that these reflect some more general asymmetry of the body touching upon many organ systems. When the asymmetry of the human brain is considered, for instance, we cannot rule out the possibility that unequal development of the two sides of the brain follows other asymmetries, such as the position of the heart, which could itself cause the unequal rate of blood flow reported for the two cerebral hemispheres. The evidence for brain asymmetry has already been reviewed. Whilst it is true that the total amount of brain asymmetry is not anything like fully revealed, asymmetry is still something which needs to be evaluated in its full extent.

The question has to be raised as to the significance which attaches to asymmetry in evolution. Nature can come to the solution of her problems in a number of different and sometimes seemingly unrelated ways. Brain asymmetry is no exception to this. The range of cerebral asymmetry is wide, including gross anatomical asymmetry as well as subtle functional differences. Some of the asymmetries could be mere accidents of nature, perpetuated only because they remained neutral with respect to the question of survival. Others, perhaps giving an additional power to the brain, fostered survival and hence became incorporated as part of the standard equipment of the brain for that species.

The problem as I see it is for the brain to bring together into one working harmonious whole the contribution from its respective functioning parts. In an organism driven by its environment the bilateral brain may suffice to guide and control behaviour irrespective of any overriding communication between the two sides. With increasing sophistication and an enhanced capacity to abstract mental function away from stimulus bound behaviour the question of overall control and the production of a unitary output becomes a more important issue. There are several mechanisms by which conflict between competing structures and resolution towards one central course of action could be produced. Each separate half of the bilateral brain could act as its own determinant. If the decisions from the two sides converged, as for the most part they would, there need be no problem. Conflict and vacillation could, however, exert some toll on the survival of the animal. Another solution would be to allocate to one side the ultimate command over action. I believe that it is to this that we can attribute most known asymmetries of the brain, i.e. the development of a system of control responsible for gathering information from both sides but ultimately generating the commands for action out of the one brain location. Here, asymmetry represents the search by the brain for unity of control despite the fact that the bilateral structure gives other important advantages.

In some cases the major resolution is an anatomical one. Corballis and Morgan (1978) suggest, for example, that an underlying growth process is the feature which distinguishes the difference between the right and the left hemisphere for man. During brain development the left hemisphere has an early growth advantage and therefore it reaps the fruits of the early developer, whereas the right hemisphere shows developmental lag and suffers the consequences which equally follow from this. This is an interesting and important idea which brings together a great deal of diverse factual information from many areas of brain science concerned with this problem. If this view is correct the human brain solves its identity crisis quite early on by virtue of the differential patterns of growth, and so integrity and unity is superimposed on the bilateral brain of man as a part of the natural course of development.

Much recent history of the brain can be seen as directed to bringing the lateral structures into a full integrated relationship. Although there is evidence to suggest that brain size for man has very recently been on the increase, it is a fact that for millions of years of human history the cranial vault remained almost totally unchanged in size, thus fixing the space to be given to the development of the brain. With this gross restriction on the expansion in terms of absolute size, severe restrictions were placed on the further advancement of the brain. One area of advancement was possible none the less and that lay in structures which could fill the gaps between the two hemispheres. It is here in the corpus callosum and the other neocortical commissures that we see a major recent evolutionary advance in the structure of the brain. The contribution of these structures to mental life is an important one. It is commonly argued that the corpus callosum lacks cell bodies and contains only white fibres and therefore its function must be merely as a conducting tract to carry information between one hemisphere and the other. The split-brain research (see Chapter 9 of this volume) shows that it does indeed fulfil a major function of this sort. As regards the integration between the bilateral systems of the brain, however, it is clear that in the development of these neocortical systems we witness a new and important solution to the problem of the unification of widely separate and rather diverse mechanisms of the brain. The callosum represents an important achievement in the process of integration.

Does the callosum do anything except transmit information from one side to the other? Despite the fact that it consists solely of white fibres there is some case to be made out for considering it to have some other functions. Because the cell bodies lie at either side within the fabric of the hemispheres themselves, this extended system could be considered a third unit of neocortex lying between the other two and serving, through the process of cross-talk and decision, to exercise an overriding control over functions expressed at either side. This view would put the callosum as less of a connection and rather more as an instrument of decision; certainly as one of the major integrating networks exercising the principles of control within the brain. The development of neocortical control via the callosum therefore has to be classed together with asymmetry as one of the major attempts of nature to create unity out of the working of the disparate parts of the brain. (For an earlier discussion of the advantages of a double brain, which expands some of the points made in this section, see Dimond (1972).)

Lateralized function in man

To illustrate current knowledge of lateralized function in man it is proposed to deal here mainly with the split-brain condition. The reason is not that important knowledge does not exist elsewhere (e.g. Kimura, 1973) but rather that split-brain work is perhaps more circumscribed than the rest and arguably it forms a core of work from which much else is derived. For reviews of this area see Beaumont (1978), Dimond (1972), Dimond and Beaumont (1974) and Sperry (1974).

Bogen and Vogel in 1962 described how they sectioned the

corpus callosum to treat an epileptic patient who had been having seizures for more than ten years, and who had continued to worsen despite extensive medication. Following this a considerable improvement was observed. It was reported that five and a half years after surgery the patient had not had a single generalized convulsion, that the level of medication had been reduced, and that it had been possible to obtain an overall improvement in behaviour and well-being. A new series of patients are now under study (Gazzaniga, 1977) and these patients offer an opportunity to extend and confirm much of the earlier work as well as to highlight some important differences.

The split-brain patient for example when tapped on a finger on one hand may be unable to transfer the information across and so cannot indicate with the corresponding finger of the opposite hand where he had been tapped. What the patient sees in one visual field may be available only to one hemisphere. Thus when a pattern is flashed to either the right or the left visual field the patient can identify the stimulus with his left hand only if it appears in the left visual field. When the pattern is flashed to the right visual field the patient can identify the stimulus with his right hand or verbally. It appears clear that each disconnected hemisphere has the capacity to perceive, to remember and to learn, and that the experienced contents of one hemisphere are not of necessity the same as those of the other.

Important differences exist between the capacities and specializations of the two sides of the brain, particularly the predominant localization of linguistic abilities in the left hemisphere of most individuals (Dimond, 1972; Gazzaniga, 1967; Geschwind, 1972; Kimura, 1973; Sperry, 1968). Constructional tasks involving a large spatial component are performed more proficiently by the left hand (right hemisphere) than by the right hand (left hemisphere). The right hemisphere appears to be more proficient generally in visual-spatial tasks including copying diagrams and assembling blocks. The right hemisphere has an intellect capable of performing geometry, matching figures to their parts and an overall proficiency in dealing with spatial problems. As regards language the first indications were that the right hemisphere possessed only a rudimentary capacity to speak, perhaps little more than a few expletive words. The first indications also suggested that it had little comprehension of spoken or written language, although this view has changed over the years and a greater level of attainment is now attributed to it. As regards the differential perceptual capacities, a widely held belief is that the right hemisphere operates on a gestalt basis with a capacity for ready visualization and immediate grasp of spatial relationships.

Something of this may be seen when the patient is presented with a chimeric stimulus test in which each hemisphere receives a different and conflicting pattern. The pattern received on the right hemisphere is usually given priority in this circumstance, and this is the one chosen as correct for matching purposes. The same holds true for chimeric faces, (that is, faces composed of two different half pictures, each flashed to separate hemispheres.) Again the half face flashed to the right hemisphere (left visual field) is the one usually matched to the original whole face – unless naming of the face is required and then the left hemisphere has the advantage. This effect appears to be part of an advanced perceptual capacity of the right hemisphere which generally confers an advantage when a face stimulus is used for recognition.

One striking and undeniable feature of the performance of the left hemisphere of the split-brain person is the facility which exists for speech. The first patient tested by Bogen and Vogel showed language lateralization to a marked degree. He could describe the events which happened on the right side of his body but not those on the left. He could describe objects seen in the right visual field but when questioned about objects in the left visual field he often appeared surprised and claimed that he saw nothing. The patient could identify objects on the left side by pointing, however, but like the deaf mute he could not say what they were. I have recently retested a patient bilingual in Spanish and English who spoke both languages fluently. Both languages were available for the description of objects or stimuli in the right visual field, but neither was available for the description of objects in the left visual field. It is clear from this simple experiment that speech in both languages emanates from the same hemisphere (the left) and that presumably the mechanisms for both languages were laid down on that side. This simple demonstration dispenses with the notion that the bilingual makes use of separate hemispheres for the two languages.

Whilst speech and language can be remarkably preserved in split-brain patients there are none the less some unusual features. One of these is the stereotyped nature of much of what the patient says. It is a surprising experience to revisit these patients after two years to find many of them saying almost exactly the same things, and in a virtually identical manner as on a previous visit. This restricted recycling of the mental content of the left hemisphere obviously relates in part to a defect of memory (none of the patients recalled having seen the investigator previously for example) yet time stands still not only because of poor memory but rather because the same thoughts, the same mental content, are still circulating in much the same way.

Yet another feature of language which appears to apply to all the patients studied is that speech somehow appears to lack the quality of an essential interaction. The generative productive capacity is present but the speech emitted is often devoid of genuine inter-action with the situation. This feature is difficult to describe. It is as if a radio had been switched on. Speech is produced but it is somehow mechanical and unempathic. The conclusion I reached after the study of these patients is that whilst a remarkable preserva-tion of language does occur, even to the extent of maintaining the structure of two languages in the bilingual patient, there is never-theless some qualitative loss.

The part played by the right and the left hemisphere in the control of emotion is an important topic (Dimond and Farrington, 1977). Evidence now indicates a radical division of the experienced emotional content of the two sides of the brain. When, for example, sodium amytal is administered to the left or the right hemisphere to discover where speech is lateralized for the purpose of preserving it after neurosurgery, different emotional responses may occur. When the dominant hemisphere (usually the left) is inactivated it is reported that a depressive type of response is produced whereas inactivation at the opposite side produces an euphoric or maniacal reaction. Brain damage affecting one side of the brain could similarly be expected to release the other hemisphere and enable it to express more fully the nature of the emotions it contains. It is interesting to note therefore that patients with a preserved left hemisphere show behaviour in which jokes, puns, mockeries and disinhibition figure prominently. This suggests that the left hemisphere is the home of the lateralized emotions of humour and euphoria now released from the control of the darker emotions at the other side. In split-brain man also speech is usually euphoric. It is common for the patient to make quips and jokes, again indicating that the lighter aspect of the affec-tive state comes from the left hemisphere.

Farrington and I have reported studies of the emotional vision of the two sides of the brain in normal subjects when each hemisphere sees separately, via a contact lens system, a film designed to provoke an emotional response. The strength of the response is measured by changes in the subjects' heart rate. All films seen on the right hemisphere with the exception of a travel film were judged as more horrific than those seen in free vision or on the left hemisphere. The film of a surgical operation provoked the greatest heart-rate change when seen on the right hemisphere whilst a cartoon provoked the greatest heart-rate change when seen on the left hemisphere. We believe that these results show that unpleasant triggers to experience produce a genuinely enhanced response from the right hemisphere thereby suggesting that it is the right hemisphere which bears responsibility for the darker, more painful aspects of human emotion. The presence of an alternative emotional vision within the nervous system, however, is controlled by some kind of cerebral dominance because the emotional response of free vision is in all respects similar to that of the left hemisphere. Nevertheless I feel that the presence of an alternative emotional vision in the right hemisphere is important, even if its process of evaluation is suppressed for the control of everyday behaviour.

The disconnected left hemisphere certainly contains its own mechanisms for laughter and humour. It is more difficult though to demonstrate that it is deprived of those darker (depressive) emotions that are believed to characterize the emotional life of the right hemisphere. On split-brain patient, however, provided a striking natural example of this deficiency. He had recently received the news that his mother was suffering from a severe illness and would shortly die. On greeting one of the investigators he introduced the subject by saying that 'something funny' had just happened. During his account of the illness the patient displayed no verbal hint of sadness. The striking thing was the voice and what the patient said. The voice regarded the matter as one of humour more than sadness. It may be that this is how the young Californian would talk about a touching event in the family – an attempt at bravura even in the face of great personal sadness. To the onlooker, however, it appeared more as an incongruity of affect – a brain talking about the deeper emotions but using the vocabulary of humour to do so. This may be an isolated, untypical example but it did seem that the left hemisphere proceeds on a broadly euphoric basis using the language of humour and laughter whatever the other emotion.

This is presumably because that is what the left hemisphere is largely programmed to do, and that is the language which comes out of it for self-expression. Although the patients differ considerably from one another in the degree to which the deeper emotions appear to be disconnected from speech, it is certainly the case that the left hemisphere is characteristically light-hearted and possessed of humour. The way in which speech achieves contact with and so can express deeper emotions is something that requires further investigation.

There are a number of observations which suggest that the split-brain person may experience certain difficulties in the attentional sphere. Something of the incapacity to sustain attention has been observed for example on tests of motor function. The patient performing a task quite competently over a period of perhaps ten to fifteen minutes may stop, look up at the experimenter, and despite the competence of his own performance ask, 'How do I continue? What am I supposed to do now?' In an attempt to gain evidence directly relevant to the problems of the organization of attention in split-brain man I undertook some studies of vigilance in these patients (Dimond, 1976). The patient had to keep watch for signals flashed to the right or the left hemisphere. The first remarkable result of this study was the extremely poor performance of the left hemisphere. Performance was poor on both hemispheres but the left was much poorer than the right. The reason why the left behaved so badly is that it showed gaps of performance, a strange pathology of the process of consciousness, which interspersed themselves with increasing frequency as the sustained task progressed. The hemisphere appeared to pass out of contact, often for periods of 15 seconds or more. Switching to other types of lateralized signals for that hemisphere failed to activate it, but a signal switch to the right hemisphere usually resulted in a response from that side. These results suggest the powerful idea that a radical division exists in the processes of attention for the two hemispheres. The mechanisms of attention are not only divided between the two hemispheres but the attentional mechanisms at the two sides serve widely different purposes. The idea that selective attention features as a function of the left hemisphere can be supported by several lines of evidence (Dimond, 1976), and the idea that sustained attention is a quality given by the organizing functions of the right hemisphere receives unequivocal support from the results reported here.

One other aspect of these vigilance results which has not received comment as yet is the fact that vigilance performance is extremely poor in patients with total callosal section but remains as normal in those patients in whom the most posterior part of the callosum, the splenium, is preserved intact. This finding holds not only for vision but for auditory and tactual function as well. The interpretation I place on this result is that after complete splitting of the corpus callosum a consciousness circuit has been transected which in the normal brain serves to keep the individual in full communication with the world. This circuit runs between the two hemispheres and occupies a posterior position in the brain involving the splenium more than the other callosal structures.

Another phenomenon associated with consciousness which deserves further study particularly in the brain-disconnected person is that of dreaming. Galin (1974) speculated on the possibility that dreaming may be largely a function of the right hemisphere – mostly because the mental life of the dream was so typically different from that of ordinary waking activity. I recently followed this question through with six of the total commissurotomy patients of the California series. Reports of dreams were rare and mostly the patients said that they do not dream at all. One patient said that he used to have dreams but that he had not had dreams since the surgery. Another patient reported that before the operation she used to dream all the time but now she hardly dreams at all. The dreams that now she experiences are all those of the past – something that happened a long time ago.

The patients were not asked specifically about dream, content, although two described dreams with manifest sexual content, and one patient reported an unpleasant symbolic religious dream in which the devil was fighting for her soul. In so far as there appears to be a reduction of dreaming reported from the left hemisphere, splitting of the brain, it is suggested, either divides a consciousness system responsible for dreaming, or dreaming is something largely carried out by the right hemisphere and hence the dreams which occur are not available to the speaking mechanisms of the left hemisphere. One further possibility is that there are problems of recall rather than genuine difficulties in dreaming itself. One patient, for example, stated 'The best I can get out of it is no recall, because I don't remember my dreams very often when I dream. When I day-dream or dream during the day, or take a quick nap, as I do mostly on a

Saturday or Sunday, I can recall most of it then.'

Hoppe (1977) examined twelve patients after partial or total commissurectomy as well as one other patient who had undergone a complete right hemispherectomy. He reported a quantitative and a qualitative impoverishment of dreams, fantasies and symbolization, all of which he considered a manifestation of primary process thinking. Hoppe put forward the idea that the preconscious stream itself, asymbolic and imageless, is interrupted by the split of the corpus callosum. Because the feedback-free primary organizations in the right hemisphere cannot be translated by the left hemisphere, the 'private language' of dreams, fantasies and symbols is impoverished. Hoppe expresses a point of view which has gained ground in recent years that the left hemisphere plays a special part in the regulation of conscious processes whereas the right hemisphere is the home, so to speak, of preconscious mentality. I would argue, however, along the lines suggested by Zangwill (1974) that we deal here with a form of co-consciousness. The running span of subjective experience invests the mental life of both hemispheres and preconscious mentality is something different from this. According to this analysis the right hemisphere does play some special part in the production of dreams, fantasies and symbolization. In the split brain the specialized stream of consciousness which produces these is dissociated from the left hemisphere with the consequence that the left side can no longer draw on this as a part of its productive mental capacity.

In the view of the author the contribution made by the processes of dreaming to the evolution of higher mental ability and productive intelligence, the distinguishing mark of man, is that the dream provides a reservoir of internally generated images upon which the brain can draw in the solution of its mental problems. I believe that the value of these parts of mental function is that they describe for the individual not what is probable or attainable but what is a possibility. The dream in other words is no accidental epiphenome-non, it is not the system by which we relieve our daily anxieties, but rather a powerhouse of images – a central generator for the processes of intellectual function. Perhaps the simplest way to explain both the impoverishment of dream data and the fact that the left hemisphere has at least some access to dreams is to suppose that dreaming is something which originates from the consciousness-circuits of the brain and that it is associated with parts of the brain modified to produce the running span of conscious experience.

The dream in other words is part of the span of conscious experience produced by the same system which generates it in ordinary waking life. In so far as a system of this kind is presumed to span both hemispheres the disconnected left hemisphere still retains the propensity for the dream as part of its own divided consciousness-circuit. The amount of dreaming available for report is reduced because the right hemisphere contribution cannot be included. A reduction in dream reporting would thus follow simply as a natural consequence of the division of the hemispheres. Yet the evidence is not inconsistent with the idea that the right hemisphere is largely responsible for the production of dreams, although not exclusively so. It would be interesting indeed if the right hemisphere could be regarded as a source of special dream images and mental creations upon which mental life elsewhere can draw and utilize productively.

Lateralization and consciousness

Naturally with Professor Sperry making the final comment in this volume on the subject of consciousness in man it is inappropriate to dwell on this topic in detail. It is difficult, however, to come to the end of this chapter without some discussion of consciousness and the way in which it may relate to different lateralized aspects of the brain. Sperry has pointed out that consciousness is an emergent property of the universe. As life had its origin and subsequent evolution, so we may suppose consciousness originated in the cosmos and that it too has undergone its period of evolution although whether this begins and ends with man is still a matter for debate (see Chapters 7 and 9 of this volume). Indeed in its own terms the problem of the evolution of consciousness is every bit as important as that of the origin of life in the universe. It represents a central problem for the neurosciences.

The idea that consciousness is a unitary thing incapable of further analysis into component parts or subdivision is again I believe something which should not pass without challenge. There are those who support the idea of consciousness as an indissoluble unity which invests the world of mental processes. The attractiveness of this view is undeniable; yet at the same time the very elegance of the formulation should not blind us to the possibilities which exist, inherent in the analysis of its parts. For example, a great symphony is whole and indivisible as a complete experience and yet that very symphony is itself composed of separate movements, and the movements themselves are constructed out of themes and counterthemes. The total effect is created out of the individual speaking voices of the instruments of some ninety or so musicians. In line with this analysis the view I advocate is that though consciousness is special it is at the same time capable of some further analysis. Such analysis of the different lateralized components of consciousness itself allows important insights into the way consciousness is constructed. I suggest that the study of consciousness is an empirical problem and that there can be a genuine neuropsychological approach as with any other empirical problem of the brain and mind. Through the study of patients who show obvious changes in consciousness as the result of damage to different regions of the brain we can (i) build up a picture of those regions of the brain likely to be involved and (ii) carry out a functional analysis of which parts of the brain do what in contributing to the processes of consciousness themselves.

We now ask whether it is possible to analyse consciousness into its components, There are several contenders which may be put forward, though of course any listing must be regarded as provisional and in-complete. From the evidence of neuropsychological studies the following candidates suggest themselves: (1) running span of sub-jective experience; (2) dreams and dreaming; (3) relationship to the external world; (4) body awareness; (5) systems of attention and (6) self consciousness. These systems may or may not be analysable into separate entities and obviously they contribute to one whole process, but it is instructive nevertheless to ask how these themselves may fit into a schema of lateralized brain function.

In so far as consciousness can be described as the running span of subjective experience there seems every reason to suppose that each hemisphere has its own band of consciousness. If it can be accepted that splitting of the brain results in a division of consciousness between the two hemispheres and that disorders of consciousness follow the transection of the neocortical commissures, then it would follow that some part of the consciousness-circuit running between the two hemispheres is divided as a result of the surgery. If this occurs only with the loss of the posterior part of the corpus callosum (the splenium) and not in connection with surgery further forward then this suggests that the circuitry lies towards the back of the brain rather than at the front. What seems to exist is a consciousness-circuit straddling the brain but with its major components located in the hemispheres at either side. Following surgery there is a division of mental content and function which suggests that consciousness in the sense of the running span of subjective experience has been divided and that separate spheres of consciousness have now been created at each side.

The idea that there exist systems in the cortex responsible for the running span of subjective experience lying towards the back of the brain is further suggested by studies of patients with the so-called syndrome of cortical blindness (or 'blindsight', see Chapter 7 of this volume). In these patients the cortical areas for vision are destroyed rendering them blind, i.e. they have no conscious experience of vision. If however such patients are requested to guess the position of objects in their immediate environment they can, providing their eyes remain open, often do so with a fair level of success. These patients use an alternative visual system to the conscious one. It seems to me that this work can be interpreted as showing that visual cortex feeds the consciousness-system to provide vision as subjective experience. The cortically blind person probably lacks therefore a visual feed into a system for consciousness which probably lies in close proximity to the visual receiving systems located towards the back of the brain, although these sytems are to be distinguished from the visual receiving areas themselves.

Can this consciousness-circuit be further differentiated along the right-left dimension? The fact that the productive capacities of the two hemispheres are preserved at both sides, although the two are disconnected, suggests that subjective experience exists at both sides and that this is a general rather than a localized property of the system. Sustained and selective attention I suppose to be a phenomenon generated out of the circuit of consciousness, but one where evidence exists of a more specialized differentiation between the two sides; the right playing a special part in the processes of sustained attention. For dreams and dreaming also there seems to be a special component which draws extensively upon the mechanisms of the right hemisphere.

Another way in which the processes of consciousness may be diff-erentiated in the left and right hemisphere concerns those aspects which relate to consciousness of the self (see also Chapter 9 of this volume). To investigate the concept of the self and the possibility that it might be generated by the left hemisphere, as Eccles and others have suggested, I examined the reports of split-brain patients when speaking of the actions of the right as well as of the disconnected left hand. How does the speaking hemisphere regard actions generated from itself or out of the right hemisphere, over which it might have no immediate and direct control?

One patient describes some of the activities of his right and left hand thus:

> My right hand has always been under control. My right hand I've always had complete dexterity and know what to do with it – my left hand – I have to fight with it. . . . I sit on my hands a lot. If I'm reading I can hold the book in my right hand, it's a lot easier to sit on my left hand, than to hold it with both hands, than fighting it. I compensate for everything that's wrong or feels wrong. One hand that fights you. I cannot use it a lot. If I had to lose an arm I'd rather lose my left arm than my right one. The right one knows what I want it to do and it does it. The psychological effect of this is kind of weird too because you tell your hand – I'm going to turn so many pages in a book – turn 3 pages – then somehow the left hand will pick up two pages and you're at page 5 or whatever. It's better to let it go, pick it up with the right hand, and then turn to the right page. With your right hand you correct what the left has done.

There are several points to note about this patient's descriptions of the relationship between his right and left hand. The first is that the speaking hemisphere sees the right hand clearly as its own agent, the patient himself (or rather the speaking hemisphere – the *I* referred to) knows what to do with it. Already we can identify a unit of the self which consists of the left hemisphere, calls itself *I*, sees itself as the home of the person, and has a right hand which as its agent is strictly under its control. 'My left hand – I have to fight with it' – the patient here expresses the idea of a disconnection in the patterns of control and his left hand. He expresses conflict as a fight between himself and his left hand. In other words the left hand is different or operating under a locus of control which is different from 'he' himself. This is an illuminating remark about the structure of the self because the left hemisphere manifests the idea of selfhood in all that it says, and the idea is powerfully expressed that the left hemisphere not only contains the self but speaks as the self, whereas the left hand and its system of control stands as something apart from this.

If equivalence of control had been predicted between the two sides, great embarrassment could be expected on the part of the speaking hemisphere because of the interference of its opposite member. There are occasions when this occurs, as for example when the left hand turns over the pages of a book and the patient finds that he is reading the wrong page. Nevertheless examples of this kind do not distinguish behaviour all of the time. The striking fact is that the left hemisphere for the most part uses a series of techniques by which it brings everything under left hemisphere control. The patient, for example, sits on his left hand, as he picks up the book with his right hand and controls it this way. This very act alone suggests that the left hand is able to take some controlling direction which overrides the right hemisphere. This in turn suggests some process of self-direction whereby the focus of the person belongs to the left rather than to the right hemisphere. It is a long argument from the dominance of one hemisphere over the other to the argument that there is a unique self-property possessed by one hemisphere which is not shared or possessed only dimly by the other. Nevertheless, the fact that the left hemisphere for the majority of time appears to control directly or indirectly the functions of both hemispheres suggests something of the sort.

Several patients reported burning their left hand when cooking. How can it be that the left hand, capable of expressing its own independent will, can apparently be suppressed in function to the point that it gets left lying on the stove, often for several seconds at a time? Its actions exist for the most part under visual control from the left hemisphere, and thus knowledge about the hands is brought to a common hemisphere. The left arm passes out of visual control when the patient looks away to something else. These curious observations about the left hand suggest to me that a difference in volitional control exists whereby the left hemisphere contains a 'self' programmed to assume overall control of the body, and in this instance it is the left hemisphere which gives the volition for the programmed series of actions involved in cooking. In other words, it is the self-will of the left hemisphere which here prevails. It is the left hemisphere preparing food and feeding the individual, employing the left hand to assist in this by keeping it under left hemisphere observation. On occasions, however, the left hand escapes this scrutiny and it is on these occasions that the danger of burning occurs.

Another patient describes some of the things that her left hand has done in the following way:

> You wouldn't want to hear some of the things this left hand has done – you wouldn't believe it. It acts independently a lot of times. I don't even tell it to – I don't know its going to do anything. Sometimes I go to get something with my right hand, the left hand grabs it and stops it – for some reason. Then one time I was sitting down watching television, my left hand just got up and slapped me. Things – this hand is uncontrollable. It seems to have a mind of its own. Sometimes, to my dismay, it gets up and slaps me. Sometimes in the morning I wake up at a certain hour – I don't have a clock in the bedroom – I have a clock in the kitchen – and that left hand slaps me awake – boy, sometimes it gets out of hand. Look what happened – what happened was somebody slapped me. It was my left hand all the time. I was asleep, completely asleep, then all of a sudden – slap – the left hand slapped me awake. In other words I usually wake up at a certain hour just automatically – I guess I've had my rest for the night. When I've had enough sleep I wake up – but this one morning – I don't know which morning it was now – you can't pin me down on that – one morning the left hand for some reason – it was 15 minutes after 6 and usually I wake up right at 6 – Whang that left hand slapped me awake – I'm getting violent with myself. My Gosh!

The description by this patient of the condition of experiencing within herself the consequences of the division of the hemispheres raises several interesting points. First of all the account is full of humour and it was intended to be so. The account might even suggest dissociation of sleep patterns between the one hemisphere and the other. The idea of the left hand slapping the person awake suggests that the controlling mechanism of the left hand was already awake and prepared to take action. Second, there is the explicit acknowledgement from the patient that the left hand often acts independently. There is no question of the right hand acting independently. But independently from what? The left hand acts independently only from some source of intentions generated from the left hemisphere.

In this patient's description of her own condition the impression is given of a person dealing with a wayward infant that is somewhat difficult to control. Although at first the problem is approached as one of the possession of a dissident hand, immediately afterwards there comes the idea of some force, something outside. Then the idea is expressed that the left hand does not do what *she* (the person) tells it to do. This points to two important features; first, that the left hand in its waywardness stands as a separate independent force and, secondly, that it stands outside the personal identity of the patient (left hemisphere). Here we have the left hemisphere asserting itself, at least in the spoken word, as the home of the person's identity – as the individual being which she is.

This patient also provides an example of the right hemisphere interfering with the left in its programme of actions. It was the left hand which interfered with the right as it was going to grab something. Clearly there are examples where the programme from the right hemisphere predominates and the right controls the left, but usually the reverse is the case. The patient in speaking is prepared to accord 'some reason' to this action of the right hemisphere, although she wonders what it may be.

These examples all highlight one strange and important fact and that is that, although the cerebral mechanisms have been divided, the feeling generated from within the hemisphere and displayed in left hemisphere speech is one in which the essential unity of the individual is completely preserved. The examples of disconnection cited challenge this feeling but they never destroy it. Neural mechanisms have escaped from the control of the system but the left hemisphere still expresses itself as a person, essentially whole and undiminished. This appears as yet one more surprising example of the capacity on the part of the brain to restructure, on the basis of what is left after damage, a complete and whole function – or at least an internally generated feeling of completeness and essential integrity. The capacity of the brain to generate a whole person out of only an assemblage of its parts must be seen as one of the most remarkable of its achievements, displaying in doing so one of the great illusory forces of the human mind and one of the important lateral divisions of consciousness.

My conclusion is that there is a left hemisphere basis for the generative mechanisms of self and identity. Identity is expressed in all that the patient says and in what the patient does. Whether the right hemisphere also possesses a mechanism for a generative self is difficult to judge. It may, for example, recognize photographs of the person and identify in that way, but this is not what one means by the generative processes of self. That language can be used as an indispensable mechanism of self-expression is undeniable. There is probably, therefore, a particular relationship between the generative mechanisms of the self and spoken language which is used in the human species as the characteristic mode of self-expression. My belief is that if the right hemisphere contributes to this at all then its contribution is small, whereas the left hemisphere plays a large demonstrable part in the process. The split-brain patient when talking sees the part that is speaking as the source of the self. In addition there is the related question of a leading left hemisphere in cerebral dominance as well as the question of visual control by the left hemisphere over the left hand after split-brain surgery. I suggest that there is an identifiable memory system, separate in large measure from the rest, which has special reference to the self and serves it as a personal diary. What happens with respect to memory may be mirrored by other attributes. Is there, for example, a perceiving system of the self where the 'feature detectors' look inward rather than without? Is there a system which generates action out of its internal fabric and produces a unity of action out of corporate effort? We are, I submit, not totally incapable of approaching these questions at the present time.

Conclusions

In considering the plural structure of the brain and the mental life which flows from each structure the scientist has the advantage that it is actually possible to observe the effects of the separated parts of the association, to examine their independent mentality and the way they behave as separate beings. It is these separate beings which are combined back together into the total fabric which is the person. Theories of perception, information processing, vigilance and so on proceed on the basis that there is a single mechanism which underlies each process. The notion of parallel processing, however, has long been familiar to psychologists (e.g. Neisser, 1967), though I believe that insufficient attention is still paid to the possibility that diverse systems may be at work and that each simultaneously produces something different from the other. In studies of vigilance behaviour, for example, in our research we find different characteristics of vigilance on the right hemisphere from those on the left, even in the normal (Dimond, 1977). A vigilance decrement occurs in one hemisphere but not in the other. What is theory to make of this? Clearly hypotheses about such a decrement apply to one hemisphere but not the other. I believe that results of this kind undermine the fabric of much current thinking which rests its case on naïve unitarianism. The brain itself is teaching us with all the power at its command that it is a city of many happenings and doings and that for its explanation we have to think in terms of multiple mechanisms and pluralistic psychology.

The possibility of mentality outside language is one of the most important aspects of the pluralism of the brain, though it is interesting that language has the primacy that it has. Language immediately makes a claim for itself to be a prince amongst the mental processes, and to be the exclusive medium of mental function, denying often by its existence the presence of other modes of thought. The primacy of language as perceived through its own system is, I believe, responsible for the creation of two fundamental illusions. The first of these concerns the production of an illusory self. This production is on a level with the phenomenon so well known in other quarters as an active structuring of experience. The second illusion is that of the essential unity of the individual. All the evidence suggests that the brain must analyse at many levels and that its mental activity is composed of different parts, and yet whenever one argues about mental pluralism and the importance of the multi-layered approach, the fact is that the brain fails to recognize this and remains dominated by the unified strand of its own subjective experience. Despite this internally generated feeling of oneness, however, it is the analytical pluralistic approach which I believe holds out most hope for the scientific future of brain investigation.

Note

1 Some of the observations reported in this chapter were made whilst the author was in receipt of a NATO Senior Scientist Fellowship at the California Institute of Technology. I am most grateful to Professor R. W. Sperry for the opportunity to examine the split-brain patients under his care.

References

Beaumont, J. G. (1978) Split-brain studies and the duality of consciousness. In G. Underwood and R. Stephens (eds) *Aspects of Consciousness*. London: Academic Press.

Bogen, J. E. (1971) Final panel (Part iv). In W. L. Smith (ed.) *Drugs and Cerebral Function*. Springfield, Illinois: C. C. Thomas.
Bogen, J. E. and Vogel, P. J. (1962) Cerebral commissurotomy in man. Prelimary case report. *Bulletin of the Los Angeles Neurological Society 27*: 169.
Brown-Sequard, C. E. (1874) Dual character of the brain. Smithsonian Misc. Collections. The Toner Lectures, Lecture II. Smithsonian Institute, Washington D.C.
Corballis, M. C. and Morgan, M. S. (in press) On the biological basis of human laterality. *The Behavioural and Brain Sciences*.
Dewson, J. H. III, Burlingame, A., Kizer, K., Dewson, S., Kenney, P. and Pribram, K. H. (1975) Hemispheric asymmetry of auditory function in monkeys. *Journal of the Acoustical Society of America 58*: S 66.
Dimond, S. J. (1972) *The Double Brain*. Edinburgh and London: Churchill Livingstone.
Dimond, S. J. (1976) Brain circuits for consciousness. *Brain, Behaviour and Evolution 13*: 376–95.
Dimond, S. J. (1977) Vigilance and split brain. In R. Mackie (ed.) *Vigilance*. New York: Plenum Press.
Dimond, S. J. (1978) *Introducing Neuropsychology* Springfield, Illinois: C. C. Thomas.
Dimond, S. J. and Beaumont, J. G. (eds) (1974) *Hemisphere Function in the Human Brain*. London: Elek Science.
Dimond, S. J. and Blizard, D. (eds) (1977) Evolution and lateralization of the Brain. *Annals of the New York Academy of Sciences 299*. New York Academy of Sciences.
Dimond, S. J. and Farrington, L. (1977) Emotional response to films shown to the right or left hemisphere of the brain measured by heart rate. *Acta Psychologia 41*: 255–60.
Galin, D. (1974) Implications for psychiatry of left and right cerebral specialization. *Archives of General Psychiatry 31*: 572–83.
Gazzaniga, M. S. (1967) The split brain in man. *Scientific American 217* (2): 24–9.
Gazzaniga, M. S. (1977) Consistency in brain organization. In S. J. Dimond and D. Blizard (eds) Evolution and lateralization of the brain. *Annals of the New York Academy of Sciences 299*: 415–23.
Geschwind, N. (1972) Language and the brain. *Scientific American 226* (4): 76–83.
Geschwind, N. and Kaplan, E. (1962) A human cerebral disconnection syndrome. *Neurology 12* (10): 675–85.
Harnad, S., Doty, R. W., Goldstein, L., Jaynes, J. and Krauthamer, G. (eds) (1977) *Lateralization in the Nervous System*. New York: Academic Press.
Hoppe, K. D. (1977) Split brains and psychoanalysis. *Psychoanalytical Quarterly 46*: 220–44.
Jackson, J. H. (1874) On the duality of the brain. In J. Taylor (ed.) *Selected Writings of John Hughlings Jackson*, Vol. II. London: Hodder and Stoughton.
Kimura, D. (1973) The asymmetry of the human brain. *Scientific American 228* (3): 70–8.

Levy, J. (1977) The mammalian brain and the adaptive advantage of cerebral asymmetry. In S. J. Dimond and D. Blizard (eds) Evolution and lateralization of the brain. *Annals of the New York Academy of Sciences 299.*

Neisser, U. (1967) *Cognitive Psychology.* New York: Appleton-Century Crofts.

Nottebohm, F. (1977) Asymmetries in neural control of vocalization in the canary. In S. Harnad, R. W. Doty, L. Goldstein, J. Jaynes and G. Krauthamer (eds) *Lateralization in the Nervous System* New York: Academic Press.

Oppenheimer, J. (1977) Studies of brain asymmetry. In S. J. Dimond and D. Blizard (eds) Evolution and lateralization of the brain. *Annals of the New York Academy of Sciences 299.*

Sperry, R. W. (1964) The great cerebral commissure. *Scientific American 210* (1): 42–52.

Sperry, R. W. (1968) Hemisphere deconnection and unity in conscious awareness. *American Psychologist 23*: 723–32.

Sperry, R. W. (1974) Lateral specialization in the surgically separated hemispheres. In F. O. Schmitt and F. G. Worden (eds) *The Neurosciences Third Study Program.* Cambridge, Mass.: M.I.T. Press.

Wigan, A. L. (1844) *The Duality of Mind. A New View of Insanity.* London: Longman, Brown, Green and Longman.

Witelson, S. (1977) Anatomic asymmetry in the temporal lobes: its documentation, phylogenesis and relationship to functional asymmetry. In S. J. Dimond and D. Blizard (eds) Evolution and lateralization of the brain. *Annals of the New York Academy of Sciences 299.*

Young, J. Z. (1962) Why do we have two brains? In V. B. Mountcastle (ed.) *Interhemispheric Relations and Cerebral Dominance.* Baltimore: Johns Hopkins University Press.

Zangwill, O. L. (1974) Consciousness and the cerebral hemispheres. In S. J. Dimond and J. G. Beaumont (eds) *Hemisphere Function in the Human Brain.* London: Elek Science.

9 Consciousness, freewill and personal identity[1]

R. W. Sperry

Two special properties of the brain not found in other natural systems, as far as we yet know, have always been notoriously difficult for science to deal with – even in principle. The first of these, of course, is conscious awareness, that will-o'-the wisp that science cannot find, cannot demonstrate, measure or work with and, in most cases, something just the basic nature of which we have been unable to conceive satisfactorily or even imagine. How the brain mechanisms generate subjective conscious experience continues to pose the number one problem for brain research and one of the most truly mystifying unknowns remaining in the whole of science (see also Chapters 7 and 8 of this volume).

The second brain property that science finds particularly troublesome is freewill. Science is concerned with causal relations and can hardly work out the natural laws, predictions and understanding of a system that fails to obey the principles of lawful causation. One of the earliest rules for animal behaviour stated that when rigorous conditions are established in which all sensory input can be strictly controlled, one may predict for any measured stimulus that an animal will respond 'as it damn pleases'. This was widely referred to back in the 1930s as the 'Chicago Law of Behaviour' – or, in Chicago, as the 'Harvard Law'.

It is curious and perhaps not entirely coincidental that these two brain properties that science finds so unaccountable are commonly considered by practically all of us to be the two most important and most treasured of all our brain faculties. In approaching some of the critical problems involved I turn first to related observations concerning personal identity and the unity of the self. It has been argued by Anderson (1974) that if one can have two co-conscious entities occupying the same cranium concurrently, as in commissurotomy (split-brain; see chapter 8 of this volume) subjects, and if two or more different persons can occupy the same body successively, as in multiple personality or fugue states, it follows logically that it is no longer correct to identify a 'person' or 'self' as being correlated one-to-one with a body. The concepts and definitions of 'person', 'self' and related terms need accordingly to be refined more precisely in terms of the critical brain states involved. Such definitions become important for medicolegal issues concerning, for example, comatose, anencephalic or severely deranged mental conditions, in evaluating donors for vital organ transplants, in dealing with different stages in foetal development, etc.

An interesting position in regard to the concept of 'personal identity' has been taken by Puccetti (1973, 1976) and Bogen (1969) who infer that each hemisphere must have a mind of its own – not only after brain bisection but in the normal intact state as well; a conclusion apparently accepted also by De Witt (1975) with the qualification that only the left cerebral member has self-awareness and is therefore qualified as a person. The argument goes like this: if cutting the cross-connections between the hemispheres leaves two co-conscious minds, and if surgical removal of a whole hemisphere, that is, hemispherectomy, leaves one conscious person or self, regardless of which hemisphere is removed, then there must have been two present to start with. Puccetti contends that we are, therefore, all of us, really a compound of two conscious persons that coexist in the normal brain, one based in each hemisphere, and that this goes undetected when the commissures are intact and the normally conjoined hemispheres work in perfect synchrony. A similar proposal regarding the inherent duality of mind was made back in 1844 by Wigan (see Zangwill, 1974). Again one is impressed with the need for sharpening definitions of mind, person, self and related concepts. Regardless of terminology, however, the question of whether the normal intact brain contains only one unified realm of conscious awareness or alternatively maintains two separate conscious systems, or minds, one centred in each hemisphere, poses a rather clear dichotomy that should be subject eventually to a definite empirical answer.

My own position on this question has been a relatively conventional one. I see consciousness and the conscious self as being normally single and unified, mediated by brain processes that typically involve and span both hemispheres through the commissures. This interpretation implies, first, that the fibre systems of the brain mediate the stuff of conscious awareness as well as the switching mechanisms, synaptic interfaces or other interaction sites of the grey matter. Second, that the fibre cross-connections between the hemispheres are not different in this respect from fibre systems within each hemisphere. Third, this interpretation is based on a functionalist theory of consciousness that goes back to the early 1950s (Sperry, 1952) in which the subjective unity in conscious experience along with other subjective effects is ascribed not so much to corresponding spatio-temporal unity in neural activity or to other isomorphic or topological correspondence but rather to the operational or functional effects in brain dynamics. What counts in determining subjective meaning on these terms is the way a given brain process works in the context of cerebral organization. Subjective unity is accordingly conceived in terms of organizational and functional relations which in turn leads to the idea of a functional (thus causal) impact (see Sperry, 1976).

When I tried to put some of these threads together back in the mid-1960s, I found to my initial consternation (as well as that of immediate colleagues) that what seemed to be emerging was a conceptual formula for the way that conscious mind could move matter in the brain and exert causal influence in the direction and control of behaviour – in direct contradiction, of course, to the central founding precepts of behaviourism and of twentieth-century scientific materialism generally, and contrary to everything that we had always been taught and believed. Since the initial statement of these concepts (Sperry, 1965), however, their influence has been apparent with respect particularly to subjectivist approaches in behavioural science. As long as it remained inconceivable that phenomena of conscious experience could affect the course of brain events, those disciplines in psychology that rely on introspective reports of subjective experience, including the clinical, humanist, cognitive and related schools, continued to be put down in dominant behaviourist thinking as something less than scientific. Once a credible conceptual model for psychophysical interaction became recognized, wherein mental phenomena as top-level controls were neither identical with nor reducible to neural events, the scientific status of consciousness and of the subjective approach underwent a change. Terms like 'mental imagery' and visual, verbal or auditory 'images' and all forms of inner thought, motivation and feeling now became more acceptable as explanatory constructs. After more than fifty years of being strictly avoided on behaviourist principles, such subjective terms have recently exploded into wide usage (Pylyshyn, 1973) in a change variously referred to as the 'cognitive' (Dember, 1974), 'humanist' or 'third' (Matson, 1973) revolution in psychology. Meantime in the mind-brain controversy, mentalists, dualists and psychophysical interactionists have suddenly begun to reappear in force, after having been essentially silent and invisible for decades.

It is not critical at this stage that the new interpretation lacks any firm proof. No proof is available, either, for the behaviourist-materialist position. Just the fact that a scientifically possible explanatory model for psychophysical interaction is conceivable has been sufficient in itself to release the long pent-up subjectivist pressures.

At the same time, more peripheral movements leaning towards the mystical and supernatural have also been bolstered secondarily in this recent mentalist upsurge, including parapsychology. Actually no direct support for these latter can be found in our present mind-brain model. If anything, the current interpretation – in which conscious experience becomes a systemic property of and functionally tied to the physical brain process (see below) – makes less likely than ever the possible occurrence of mental telepathy, psychokinesis, precognition and other so called psi phenomena. Nor can the current view be said to encourage hopes for the existence of any separate, non-physical realm of conscious mind or spirit divorced from matter. In other words the current swing away from traditional materialism does not carry us all the way back to dualistic or supernatural concepts but represents, rather, an intermediate compromise within which aspects of both classic physicalist and mentalist doctrine are fused in a new combination.

Without attempting here to review in detail these conceptual developments let me just restate briefly that, in our current interpretation of consciousness, subjective awareness is conceived to be a functional property of neural events generated at top levels in the brain hierarchy. The emergent (functional) properties are conceived to have causal consequences in cerebral activity just as emergent properties commonly do elsewhere. The regulative control role of conscious experience is seen to be based largely in the universal power of any system as a whole over its parts. Mental phenomena built of neural events are conceived to act as dynamic entities in brain organization interacting at their own level in brain function. As high-level dynamic entities, the mental processes control their component biophysical, molecular, atomic and other subelements in the same way, for example, that the organism as a whole controls the fate of its separate organs and cells or just as the molecule as an entity carries all its component atoms, electrons and other subatomic parts through a distinctive time-space course in a chemical reaction. An expanded description of this holistic or entitative type of causal control is presented by Pols (1971).

As is the rule for part-whole relations, a mutual interaction between the neural and the mental events is indicated; the brain physiology determines the mental effects, as generally agreed, but the neurophysiology is at the same time reciprocally governed by the higher subjective properties of the enveloping mental operations, as these interact at their own level and prevail upon subsidiary events in brain dynamics. A full causal account of brain function is thus not possible in purely neurophysiological or biophysical terms that do not include these higher, yet-to-be-described mental processes with their subjective pattern properties different from the neural events *per se*.

By way of illustration, if one could render the nerve impulse and related glial activity X-ray opaque or radiant and then take fluoroscopic-like pictures of the cerebral turbulence for different kinds of conscious brain events, one might be able in time to begin to describe the critical differences that are responsible, for example, for auditory as opposed to visual or tactual sensation and later to go into further intramodal refinements describing the processing differences involved in seeing red versus green or a triangle versus a square, etc. These conscious processes, as entities, have never been described, and the objective descriptions are still far out of reach. When the objective account becomes available we will have both the objective and subjective descriptions, but the subjective effect, on these terms, should be understandable and inferable from the objective description, because the subjective meaning depends on how the brain process, as a dynamic entity, works in the going context of brain activity (Sperry, 1952). The basic organizational features involved are assumed to be genetically determined in very large part.

The foregoing combines important features of both classic dualistic mentalism and monistic materialism. It is mentalistic in that the contents of subjective mental experience are recognized as important aspects of reality in their own right, not to be identified with the neural events as these have heretofore been conceived nor reducible to neural events. Further, the subjective mental properties and phenomena are posited to have a top-level control role as causal determinants (Sperry, 1976). On these terms mind moves matter in the brain. Not only can subjective mind no longer be ignored in science; it becomes a prime control factor in explanatory models. In former theories of consciousness at all acceptable to science, consciousness has been so defined that the causal march of brain mechanisms would proceed the same, whether it is accompanied by subjective experience or not. This is not the case in the present model.

At the same time, the current view can be called materialistic, in that the subjective phenomena as functional properties of brain activity are built of neural events and therefore always tied, as emergent properties, to the physical brain with all its anatomical and physiological constraints. The classic definitions of dualism and monism hardly apply, however, and mentalism is no longer synonymous with dualism. It has seemed preferable to describe the new position as mentalist and monist (Sperry, 1965) reserving dualism for concepts that allow for a separate existence of conscious experience apart from the functioning brain.

This mind-brain reformulation brings important logical implications also for the interpretation and outlook regarding freewill. The causal sequence of brain events leading to and determining a given voluntary act or decision no longer is conceived to be restricted to a series of neurophysicochemical activities. The emergent subjective mental properties of these physical processes, as described above, must also be taken into account and included among the controlling causal determinants. This introduces new degrees and qualities of freedom into the brain's decision-making process, lifting it above the mechanistic, physicalistic kind of determinism envisaged in classical behaviourist, stimulus-response or materialist doctrine. For example, one's subjective desire to do this or that, along with other subjective feelings and motivations and subjective values of all kinds, plus the whole range of cognitive mental experience, may now, *per se*, influence the progression of brain events as directive causal factors. As dynamic, holistic properties, the subjective factors are not reducible to, or identifiable with, their neural constituents or as parallelistic correlates of these. In any decision to act, these conscious mental phenomena override and supersede the component physiological and biophysical events involved in the causal progression of brain activity.

A given volitional choice may depend additionally on things like the memory and the mental perspective acquired by the subject (and any consultants) over a span of many decades preceding the decision. Data from the information store of one or more libraries may be called on and funnelled into the brain code sequence that leads to the given choice. Even factors like the predicted long-term future consequences of the various alternative choices being contemplated may be included proactively in this vast vortex of cerebral factors that governs the final decision to act. Compared with the kinds of determinism that science deals with in other systems, the degree and levels of freedom in the operations of the human brain clearly set the brain and mind of man apart with the dignity of an apex post in the universe, far above all other known systems in terms of its ability to choose and to control a course of events.

Even so, one may object that this leaves our brain's decisions nevertheless all, in a sense, determined, even though at this higher, more complex mental level. We are still caught in the web of a deterministic universe and have to do what we do. Having *degrees* of freedom, in other words, does not quite make for *complete* freedom from causal control. The answer here is that complete freedom from causation would mean behaviour based purely on chance, on caprice and would result in meaningless chaos. What one wants of freewill is not to be totally freed from causation, but, rather, to have the kind of control that allows one to determine one's own actions according to one's own wishes, one's own judgement, perspective, cognitive aims, emotional desires and other mental inclinations. This, of course, is exactly what is provided in our current interpretation.

I have already stated my belief that the organizational features of the brain which give rise to conscious processes are in large part genetically determined. If this is true then consciousness must be subject to the evolutionary process. From the standpoint of functional control, one may ask what benefits precisely are conferred by the introduction in evolution of subjective conscious effects? Thinking in regard to this question is still preliminary and speculative along lines like the following: consider the tactical difference between responding to the world directly and responding to inner conscious representations of the outside world. Wherever displacements in time or in space are advantageous, as, for example, in mental recall, in thinking and in the formation of anticipatory sets, the use of inner representations has indispensable organizational advantages (see Chapter 7 of this volume). The real world can hardly be manipulated as can inner images. Responses involving perceptual constancies in shape, size, position, etc. would seem also to be more effectively managed through the use of inner representations. Further, the employment of implicit trial-and-error responses to inner mental models and the avoidance thereby of overt response commitments, with possible errors in the real world, is a central rationale in the evolution of thinking.

The development of an inner subjective world may thus be viewed broadly as part of the evolutionary process of freeing behaviour from its initial primitive stimulus-bound condition, providing increasing degrees of freedom of choice and of originative central processing. The subjective effects have additional advantages in the driving and directing of behaviour as motivational elements and as positive and negative reinforcers. It is difficult to conceive an efficacious motivational system without subjective properties like pain, pleasure, hunger, etc. These subjective effects evolve into controlling ends in themselves in much of human behaviour.

Conscious experience may be conceived as a rather distinct entity built into brain organization and expressly designed for specific functional effects, as opposed to viewing it as a general pervasive property of complex neural integration. There is reason to believe it is present in the higher brain centres but not in the spinal cord, for example, or lower brain stem, and probably not in the cerebellum, either. The commissurotomy evidence indicates that the system for inner conscious representations in primates and cats, at least, is confined mainly to the cerebral hemispheres proper and the upper brainstem. We assume it to be rather diffusely represented within the forebrain but by no means extending throughout all neural activity at forebrain levels. On the input side of the conscious system, a great deal of sensory processing is completed automatically and unconsciously. The integrations required for constancy effects like those for perceived position in space during head, eye and body movements, or for the union of monocular two-dimensional patterns into novel three-dimensional percepts, or the processing of elemental auditory sounds into perceived speech, etc. are extremely complex neural functions but appear to be processed without conscious mediation. Similarly, on the output side, most or all of the complicated processing required to translate conscious aims, percepts and volitional intent into appropriate motor-behaviour patterns also takes place automatically and unconsciously. The intricate arrays of requisite muscle-contraction patterns involve a complexity of neural control that goes far beyond the ability of the conscious mind to understand and direct. This is another reason to identify the conscious properties with the relatively simple holistic features rather than with the whole intricate inframechanism of brain processing.

Though representing a rather small fraction of the total brain activity in physiological terms, the conscious properties are of prime importance from the organizational standpoint. For example, the laying down, storage, cataloguing and retrieval of memories seem to proceed very largely on the basis of their holistic conscious properties rather than those of the neuronal inframechanisms. Most higher brain processing can be viewed as being designed for, and directed towards the generation, maintenance or expression of aspects of conscious awareness. Older stimulus-response and central-switchboard concepts of brain organization that arose out of spinal cord physiology and were congenial to behaviourist interpretation may be replaced by a model in which the brain is seen to be organized as a decision-making control system monitored with value priorities and in which conscious phenomena confer certain operational advantages over and above those obtainable in systems that lack consciousness.

Note

1 This chapter contains material first published in *Perspectives in Biology and Medicine* (1976) *20* (1): 9, 12–15 and *The Journal of Medicine and Philosophy* (1977) *2* (2): 115–16, 121–2, selected by the editors. We are grateful to the University of Chicago Press for permission to use extracts from the original articles.

References

Anderson, S. L. (1974) On the Problem of Personal Identity. Ph.D. dissertation, University of California, Los Angeles.

Bogen, J. E. (1969) The other side of the brain. II. An appositional mind. *Bulletin of the Los Angeles Neurological Societies 34*: 135–62.

Dember, W. N. (1974) Motivation and the cognitive revolution. *American Psychologist 29*: 161–8.

De Witt, L. (1975) Consciousness, mind and self: the implications of the split-brain studies. *British Journal for the Philosophy of Science 26*: 41–7.

Matson, F. W. (1973) Humanistic theory: the third revolution in psychology, In P. Zimbardo and C. Malach (eds) *Psychology for our Times*. Glenview, Illinois: Scott, Foresman, 19–25.

Pols, E. (1971) Power and agency. *International Philosophical Quarterly 11*: 293–313.

Puccetti, R. (1973) Brain bisection and personal identity. *British Journal for the Philosophy of Science 24*: 339–55.

Puccetti, R. (1976) The mute self: a reaction to De Witt's alternative account of the split-brain data. *British Journal for the Philosophy of Science 27*: 65–73.

Pylyshyn, Z. W. (1973) What the mind's eye tells the mind's brain: a critique of mental imagery. *Psychological Bulletin 80*: 1–24.

Sperry, R. W. (1952) Neurology and the mind-brain problem. *American Scientist 40*: 291–312.

Sperry, R. W. (1965) Mind, brain and humanist values. In J. R. Platt (ed.) *New Views on the Nature of Man*. Chicago: University of Chicago Press.

Sperry, R. W. (1976) Mental phenomena as causal determinants in brain function. In G. Globus, G. Maxwell and I. Savodnik (eds) *Consciousness and the Brain*. New York: Plenum Publishing Corp.

Zangwill, O. L. (1974) Consciousness and the cerebral hemispheres. In S. Dimond and J. Beaumont (eds) *Hemisphere Function in the Human Brain*. London: Paul Elek.

Name index

Subject index